Fundamental Movement:

A DEVELOPMENTAL AND REMEDIAL APPROACH

BRUCE A. McCLENAGHAN
University of South Carolina

DAVID L. GALLAHUE
Indiana University

1978
W. B. SAUNDERS COMPANY
PHILADELPHIA • LONDON • TORONTO

W. B. Saunders Company: West Washington Square
                         Philadelphia, Pa. 19105

                         1 St. Anne's Road
                         Eastbourne, East Sussex BN21 3UN, England

                         1 Goldthorne Avenue
                         Toronto, Ontario M8Z 5T9, Canada

Library of Congress Cataloging in Publication Data

McClenaghan, Bruce A

Fundamental movement.

Bibliography: p.

Includes index.

1. Physical education for children.   2. Motor ability in
   children.   3. Physical education for exceptional children.
   I. Gallahue, David L., joint author.   II. Title.

GV443.M23   613.7'042   77–75534

ISBN 0–7216–5888–1

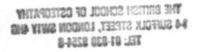

Fundamental Movement: A Developmental and Remedial Approach   ISBN   0-7216-5888-1

Last digit is the print number: 9   8   7   6   5   4   3   2   1

To Marie and Ellie, our wives, and the children of the Challengers program, from whom we have learned so much.

PREFACE

This book is directed to students, teachers, and parents concerned with the motor development and movement education of both young and exceptional children. It is designed to serve as a primary or supplemental text for courses dealing with motor development of preschool, primary, and exceptional children. The uncommon grouping of young "normal" children with exceptional children (i.e., those experiencing difficulties with cognitive, academic, and motor achievement) has been utilized because of the abundance of literature indicating that the *sequence* of acquisition of fundamental movement abilities is common for both groups although the *rate* of acquisition may differ.

Readers will appreciate the concise summarization of the current literature dealing with the acquisition and assessment of fundamental movement patterns. A readily usable observational technique for the rapid and accurate evaluation of fundamental movement patterns is an integral part of the text. It is designed to aid the teacher in accurately determining the level of motor functioning of his or her students in the categories of stability, locomotion, and manipulation.

Information obtained from the observational technique will direct the reader to specific movement experiences geared toward the child's particular level of functioning in order that these experiences may be age-appropriate and challenging, and may directly aid in the achievement of mature movement patterns.

The content of the text is divided into three sections. The first section is concerned with motor development during early childhood, with Chapter 1 serving as the introduction to the nature and use of the text. This chapter provides the reader with an overview of fundamental movement, program design, and the use of appropriate movement experiences. The second chapter is devoted to motor development during early childhood and the many early determinants of later behavior. This chapter provides the reader with valuable information for understanding the sequence of acquisition of the fundamental locomotor and manipulative abilities discussed in Chapters 3 and 4, respectively.

The second section of the book is concerned with program design and implementation. Chapter 5 presents a curriculum model for enhancing fundamental movement patterns. Methods of observing and evaluating fundamental movement are discussed in Chapter 6. This chapter presents workable, easy-to-use, and easy-to-interpret guidelines for observing and evaluating movement. Chapter 7 is concerned with methods of teaching fundamental movement. A variety of direct and indirect teaching styles are discussed with implications for both the developmental and remedial programs.

The third section of the text provides a sampling of appropriate movement experiences for enhancing fundamental movement abilities. Chapter 9 provides the reader with examples of activity ideas for developing children's physical abilities. Activities for enhancing stability, agility, flexibility, and strength abilities are presented because of their close relationship to successful performance of movement abilities. Chapters 10 and 11 present a sampling of developmental and remedial activities for improving locomotor and manipulative abilities, respectively.

Helpful appendices also provide supplemental readings for each section, a listing of inexpensive equipment for the motor development program, and an example of a commercially produced playground designed to enhance children's motor development.

The authors wish to express their gratitude to Joel Pett, who illustrated the text, to Marie McClenaghan for her typing of the manuscript, and finally to all teachers who are concerned with the total development of all children.

BRUCE A. MCCLENAGHAN
DAVID L. GALLAHUE

CONTENTS

FUNDAMENTAL MOVEMENT

SECTION CONCEPTS

1. Psychomotor development is an important factor in the total development of the young child.
2. The early childhood period is critical in the development of mature and efficient movement.
3. Numerous prenatal, natal, and postnatal factors affect a child's motor potential.
4. Fundamental movement patterns are refined in a progressive manner, and the changes that take place during this development are readily observable.

CHAPTER 1

FUNDAMENTAL MOVEMENT: AN OVERVIEW

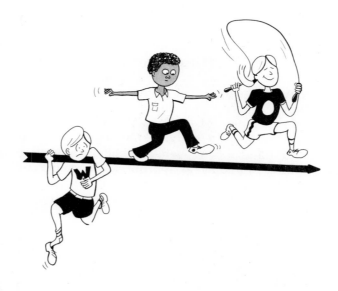

Fundamental Movement
Program Design
Movement Experiences

Interest in the motor development and movement education of young children has risen rapidly in recent years. As a result of serious study in this area, the preschool and primary grade years are no longer regarded merely as carefree and relatively meaningless years of play, games, and physical activity. Parents, educators, and psychologists all over the world are closely examining the early years as important facilitators and determinants of later cognitive, affective, and psychomotor development. The eminent developmental theorist, Jean Piaget, has sparked considerable interest in the contributions of movement to the cognitive development of children. Erik Erikson, the renowned social psychologist, strongly emphasizes the child's world of movement in his theory of psychosocial development.

Many outstanding motor development specialists in the field of physical education have demonstrated the tremendous importance of the quality and quantity of movement experiences for the balanced and complete motor development of children. Excellent work on this subject has been done by Lolas Halverson (University of Wisconsin), Carol Widule and Marguerite Clifton (Purdue University), Vernon Seafeldt (University of Michigan), Jacqueline Herkowitz (Ohio State University), Lawrence Rarick and Jack Keogh (University of California), and many others.

No longer are movement patterns of the early years looked upon as solely the product of a biological time clock (Fig. 1–1). Developmental movement experiences are considered important—in fact, necessary—for the maximum development and refinement of mature patterns of movement. The development of fundamental movement abilities is a process involving the complex interaction of both maturation *and* experience. It is a process in which we as parents and teachers can play an important role. In order to be effective, however, we must first become knowledgeable in three general areas: (1) motor development during early childhood, with particular attention to the development of fundamental locomotor and manipulative abilities; (2) program design techniques, ranging from methods of observing and evaluating fundamental movement abilities to organizing and implementing the program and applying appropriate teaching methods; and (3) appropriate developmental and remedial movement experiences for enhancing both physical and movement abilities.

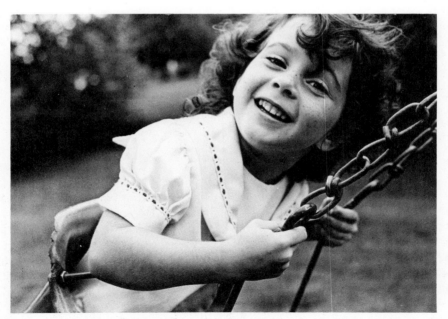

Figure 1–1 The movement patterns of early childhood are no longer regarded solely as the product of a biological time clock.

This chapter serves as an introduction to the remainder of the text. A brief overview of the contents of each of the three sections (Fundamental Movement, Program Design, and Movement Experiences) of the text is provided to familiarize the reader with the major concepts presented throughout the book.

FUNDAMENTAL MOVEMENT

The period of early childhood is a crucial time for the balanced, optimal development of the cognitive, affective, and psychomotor domains of human behavior. Because these three domains are closely interrelated, it is necessary not to omit or minimize any at the expense of another.

Too often in the past, development of psychomotor abilities has been left to chance on the assumption that maturation will take care of one's motor development. The periods of early and middle childhood provide a golden opportunity to make movement part of children's education. As well as being fun, movement is expressive, purposeful, and meaningful. It is a central way in which children learn more about themselves and their world. If left to chance, many children will *not* develop mature patterns of movement in many locomotor and manipulative activities. If these fundamental movement abilities are not developed during childhood, the chances are very slim that they will be developed and refined later in life (Fig. 1–2).

A variety of prenatal, birth, and postnatal factors influence the developmental process. The student of fundamental movement must be aware of these factors and their effect on the child's development.

Research on the development and refinement of fundamental movement abilities is relatively sparse when compared with the wealth of information we have about the skilled performer. However, a number of excellent systematic research studies have been conducted on several locomotor and manipulative patterns of movement. The literature clearly reveals that there is a developmental progression in the acquisition of fundamental movement abilities.

The locomotor movement patterns of walking, running, and jumping are discussed in detail in Chapter 3. These locomotor patterns have been selected because they represent the primary patterns upon which all other locomotor movements (hopping, skipping, leaping, and so forth) are based. They are also the only locomotor patterns that have been thoroughly researched. The manipulative patterns of throwing, catching, and kicking are included in Chapter 4 for the same reasons.

PROGRAM DESIGN

In order for knowledge of fundamental movement and the motor development of children to be of any real value, we must be able to design and implement developmentally based movement programs. One must decide on a program model that will bring order and harmony to the developmental

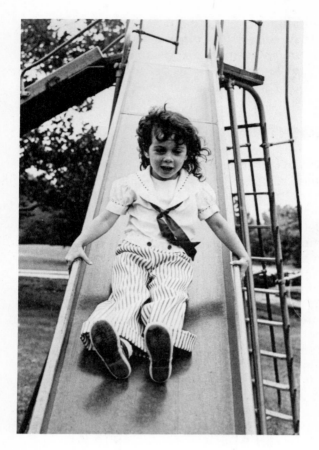

Figure 1–2 Psychomotor development is too important to be left to chance.

or remedial program. The necessary order can be ensured by choosing an approach that involves: (1) pre-program planning, (2) pre-program assessment, (3) determination of the level of cognitive and affective development of the children being taught, and (4) post-program assessment.

A crucial aspect of effective programming for children is the observation and evaluation of fundamental movement patterns. Teachers of fundamental movement should be concerned with the *qualitative assessment* as well as the *quantitative aspects* of movement. Qualitative assessment, or observation-based assessment, as it is often termed, provides the observer with valuable subjective information concerning the child's functioning. This information can in turn be used for more meaningful programming.

An informal instrument for assessing movement patterns has been developed and is presented in Chapter 6. The instrument provides a textual summary, as well as visual representations, of the developmental progression of each of the five selected patterns at the initial, elementary, and mature stages. *Movement Pattern Evaluation Sheets* are supplied for each of the five patterns. A sample *Individual Profile Sheet* is also provided and may be used as an easy-to-read summary for individual program planning. The *Class*

Inventory Summary Sheet and the *Class Ability Chart,* samples of which are included, are designed to make it possible for the teacher to chart the movement pattern development of a class or group of children. This information will enable the teacher to build the program around the actual developmental or remedial needs of individual children rather than around a hypothetical group of "average" children.

Once we have established a model for enhancing fundamental movement patterns and have utilized the observational assessment technique, it then becomes necessary to actually organize and implement the program. A variety of pre-program plans and implementation plans need to be considered. Pre-program planning involves determining the specific objectives for the particular group to be taught, with consideration given to facilities, equipment, time, staff, and instructional techniques. Implementing a successful program is the capstone of careful planning, but no movement program, no matter how carefully planned, organized, and researched, is of any real value unless effective teaching methods are employed. The mastery of various styles of teaching maximizes the effectiveness of the fundamental movement program. A variety of teaching approaches, either direct or indirect, may be utilized.

Direct methods of teaching are generally based on the command and task styles, whereas indirect teaching methods are considered exploratory and usually take the form of free exploration and guided exploration. A combination method, utilizing the best aspects of both direct and indirect methods, places the child at the center of the educational process without demanding unquestioning allegiance to any one method.

MOVEMENT EXPERIENCES

The information contained in the first two sections of the text should enable one to make knowledgeable use of the movement experiences contained in the third section. Movement experiences may be classified as those primarily intended to enhance physical abilities and those primarily intended to enhance movement abilities. The combination of the child's physical abilities and fundamental movement abilities influences his or her overall performance.

There are several kinds of physical abilities. Stability, agility, flexibility, and strength are the abilities most closely related to the performance of fundamental movement patterns. Stability is encouraged through activities on the balance beam, balance board, and inner tube. Agility is promoted through activities involving changes in the height of the body, changes in the distance the body is projected, and changes in direction. Sample activities that improve flexibility in the shoulder girdle and hip joint regions are presented. Examples of activities that promote strength in the arm and shoulder girdles, abdominal muscles, and legs are shown.

Movement abilities may be improved through various developmental or remedial experiences. Therefore, a wide variety of locomotor experiences for enhancing running, jumping, leaping, galloping, hopping, and skipping are presented. *Remedial as well as developmental activities are included for running and jumping because they are essential to the development of all other locomotor patterns. Remedial activities for throwing, catching, and kicking are also provided for the same reason.* The suggested activities are intended only to be samples of the many experiences possible. Each movement experience should contribute to the objectives of the particular lesson and the mature development of fundamental movement abilities. Moreover, each activity should be presented in a manner that is fun, exciting, and adventuresome.

CHAPTER 2

FACTORS AFFECTING MOTOR DEVELOPMENT DURING EARLY CHILDHOOD

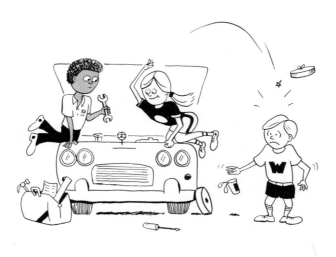

In recent years a great deal of emphasis has been placed on the role of motor development in the educational process of young children. Movement is now seen as a primary facilitator of cognitive and affective development as well as of motor development, particularly during infancy and early childhood.

The cognitive, affective, and psychomotor domains of human behavior are complexly interrelated (Fig. 2–1). Difficulty in any of these areas may adversely affect the total educational development of the child, whose cognitive, affective, and psychomotor needs vary (Fig. 2–2). Failure to develop at

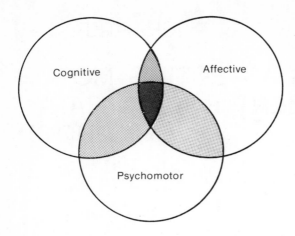

Figure 2–1 The interrelationship of the three educational domains.

a normal rate in any of the educational domains may negatively influence the rate of development in one or both of the remaining areas.

The current concern with the so-called "clumsy child" has reawakened an interest in the progressive development of motor skills in young children. *Research has indicated that although some children are delayed in the*

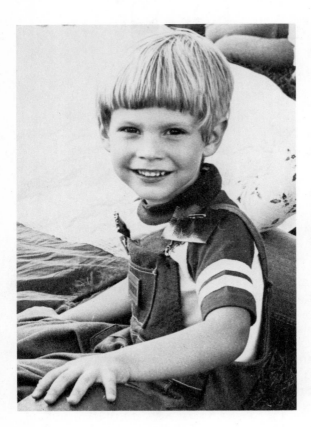

Figure 2–2 Each child has different cognitive, affective, and psychomotor needs.

acquisition of fundamental motor skills, they progress through the same developmental sequence as do normal children. Information about normal children, therefore, may be utilized in planning movement programs for young children or children who exhibit low motor ability.

From the moment of birth, motor development proceeds in an orderly manner. The newborn's movements, stimulated by the immediate environment, are largely reflexive and involuntary. As development progresses and the neurological system matures, the infant gains voluntary control over his musculature, and thus many of these reflexive movements are suppressed or inhibited. The first voluntary attempts at movement are ill-defined and gross. They appear to be random and purposeless, but actually represent a crucial information-gathering process. With time the growing child begins to integrate these ill-defined movement experiences into his ever-expanding repertoire of abilities. These movements gradually become more complex as the child learns to combine a series of individual body actions into a purposeful coordinated act or *movement pattern.* With practice and experience, these patterns become more refined, and the child begins to utilize them to perform sport-related skills. Later the adolescent begins to concentrate his efforts on refining the skills needed to perform a few specific activities on either a recreational or a competitive basis.

This chapter covers the general aspects of motor development during the early childhood period and discusses the role of fundamental movement patterns in later advanced skill development. In addition, the major prenatal, natal, and postnatal determinants that may affect a young child's motor potential are summarized.

EARLY CHILDHOOD (2 to 7)

The early childhood period is critical to the breadth and depth of motor development. In the past, most children were left on their own to develop their fundamental movement patterns. Only the movement experiences found in their everyday play activities served as the foundation for increasingly complex movements. Although the play experiences of some children are sufficiently varied to refine these patterns without the aid of planned movement experiences, it would be incorrect to conclude that most children will develop efficient and mature movement patterns without some form of instruction. Recent studies on the poorly coordinated child reinforce the contention that a significant number of children of all ages and intellectual abilities exhibit inefficient and uncoordinated movement patterns.

If a child fails to develop efficient patterns of movement during the early childhood period, he or she finds it increasingly difficult with each advancing year to acquire mature patterns. This is due primarily to three factors: (1) lack of sufficient quantity or quality of movement opportunities, (2) peer pressure, and (3) fear. This is not to say that children who develop more slowly will never achieve the mature level of functioning, but only that with

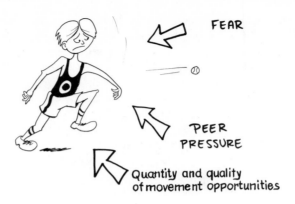

each year it becomes more difficult to develop refined fundamental movement patterns.

An example of an unskilled movement pattern commonly exhibited by older children is throwing or catching a ball. Many people, particularly females, who often have limited experiences with ball-playing during early childhood, have difficulty using a mature throwing or catching pattern. They tend to utilize an awkward arm motion and shift their weight to the wrong foot in throwing, and, when attempting to catch a tossed ball, they often exhibit an avoidance reaction with the head. The weaknesses in the throwing and catching patterns of many females, however, will probably be less evident in coming years, because increasing numbers of young girls are participating in physical activities and because there is now more positive peer group acceptance of the skilled female performer.

The fundamental movement patterns acquired during early childhood form the motor base from which more complex skills, including sports, are later developed. The degree to which children develop these fundamental abilities during early childhood often affects the ease with which they are able to achieve acceptable levels of performance in more advanced motor skills during later adolescence and adulthood. Many of these fundamental movement patterns are integrated with more complex skills and are necessary for participation in sport, dance, and recreational activities. Children who fail to develop mature and efficient movement patterns may later find it difficult to perform more complex physical skills successfully. This deficiency may have far-reaching implications for the child's ability to take part with his peers in a wide variety of play activities. Adults who have not reached the mature level in a variety of fundamental movement patterns may also have difficulty participating successfully in later recreational or competitive activities that require coordination and physical skill. The extent to which these patterns develop during early childhood depends primarily upon three factors: (1) the child's developmental potential, (2) the rate of maturation, and (3) the quality and variety of movement experiences offered.

The research dealing with the progressive development of fundamental movement patterns during early childhood tends to indicate that children attain the mature level of functioning after passing through a series of identifiable stages. In an outstanding study, Deach[15] determined whether there were, at different ages, discrete patterns of performance for the fundamental movements of throwing, catching, kicking, striking, and bouncing a ball. She demonstrated their course of development when viewed in terms of a skillful adult performance. Eighty-three boys and girls ranging in age from 34 to 83 months served as subjects. Films of each of the various performances were analyzed. The results of this study revealed that in the development of the selected patterns there was a clear progression from gross arm and leg actions to highly coordinated and integrated body actions. A three stage developmental progression, ranging from the action of a single limb to opposition of the body with total body involvement, was found in all hand-foot patterns. Similar developmental sequences have been observed by other investigators.

Within the period of early childhood, children acquire fundamental movement patterns by gradually integrating a greater number of more complex single body actions into a coordinated and refined movement pattern. The mature throwing pattern, for example, requires the performer to synchronize the body actions of the arm and hand with those of the trunk, foot, and leg. Early attempts to throw involve only an inefficient arm action centered at the elbow. With experience, the throw becomes a highly complex movement combining a number of body actions efficiently and accurately.

A review of the research on the progressive acquisition of movement patterns in young children (see Chapters 3 and 4) shows that the development of many patterns may be subdivided into a series of increasingly refined stages (Fig. 2–3). As each pattern passes through the initial, elementary, and mature stages of development, observable changes in body action take place. These changes may be used to evaluate the degree to which the

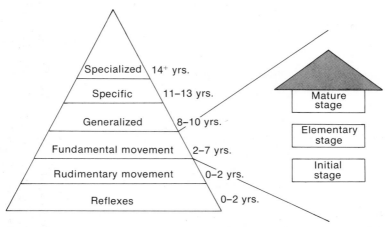

Figure 2–3 Three stage developmental progression of acquisition of fundamental movement patterns. (From Gallahue, David, Werner, Peter, and Luedke, George: *A Conceptual Approach to Moving and Learning.* Copyright © 1975 by John Wiley & Sons, Inc. Reprinted by permission of John Wiley & Sons, Inc.)

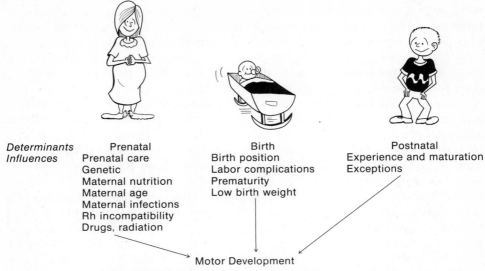

| Determinants
Influences | Prenatal
Prenatal care
Genetic
Maternal nutrition
Maternal age
Maternal infections
Rh incompatibility
Drugs, radiation | Birth
Birth position
Labor complications
Prematurity
Low birth weight | Postnatal
Experience and maturation
Exceptions |

Motor Development

Figure 2–4   Determinants of later motor development.

child has refined his fundamental movement patterns. This technique of evaluating the quality of movement is dealt with in detail in Chapter 6.

EARLY DETERMINANTS OF LATER BEHAVIOR

Throughout the developmental process, many influences may adversely affect the level of a child's motor ability. These influences may be classified as prenatal, natal, and postnatal determinants (Fig. 2–4).

PRENATAL DETERMINANTS

As early as 1913, the Children's Bureau of the United States Department of Labor, recognizing the need for informing the public about child care, published the first of a series of pamphlets on the importance of good prenatal care.[46] Each year, however, approximately half a million women fail to seek the fundamental care that is needed to reduce the risks of pregnancy.[38] Because of the numerous environmental and genetic factors that may negatively influence a child's growth and development, it is vital that expectant mothers seek professional prenatal care.

Smith[43] attempted to determine why pregnant women did not seek professional care. She found that many women believed that prenatal care was not necessary or indicated only late in pregnancy. It is estimated that each year some 250,000 American infants, or 7 per cent of all live births, are delivered with some significant birth defect. It has been estimated that 20 per cent of these defects are inherited, while 20 per cent are caused directly by environmental conditions. The remaining 60 per cent are caused by some interaction between genetic and environmental influences.[40] A significant number of these birth defects could be eliminated or minimized with proper prenatal care. The National Foundation of the March of Dimes[37] has identified "high-risk" mothers in the greatest need of prenatal care. They are:

1. Mothers under 17 or over 35 years of age
2. Mothers with metabolic disorders such as hyperthyroidism or diabetes
3. Mothers (and fathers) with family histories of any inherited disorder
4. Mothers who have previously miscarried, have given birth to an underweight or premature baby, or have a history of toxemia of pregnancy.

All cells of the human body, except the reproductive sperm and ovum, contain 23 pairs or a total of 46 chromosomes. Each chromosome contains thousands of genes that transmit genetic information from both parents, and these genes determine the genetic characteristics of the developing infant. With such a highly complex and interrelated system, errors do occur and result in genetic defects, which may be inherited basically in one of three ways.[8] One parent may be afflicted with the defect or disorder and pass it on to the child, who would have a 50 per cent chance of inheriting the impairment. Both parents, although exhibiting no impairment, may carry the recessive gene of a defect; the children then have a 25 per cent chance of inheriting the same impairment and a 50 per cent chance of being a carrier. The third method of genetic inheritance is through a faulty gene that is carried on one of the mother's X chromosomes. The mother may pass the defect on to her sons, who have a 50 per cent chance of having the defect, or she may pass the carrier state to her daughters, who have a 50 per cent chance of being a carrier. A family with a child who has this type of impairment runs only a small risk of having another child with a similar impairment. With the advent of genetic counseling and improved methods of prenatal testing, many genetic defects can now be predicted before conception or early during pregnancy.

Maternal nutrition plays an important role in the development of the fetus. The average weight gain of the expectant mother during pregnancy is approximately 24 pounds. Women who are overweight before pregnancy are often required to gain less weight, while excessively thin individuals may need to gain added weight. Some women, because of the fear that they will not be able to lose the additional weight, attempt to keep the gain as low as possible. The Committee on Maternal Nutrition[9] does not recommend a weight gain of under 14 pounds because of the adverse effect upon the fetus' birth weight and neurological development. Many expectant mothers become concerned with their diet *after* they learn they are pregnant. Studies have shown, however, that the nutritional health of the fetus depends upon the nutritional habits of the mother not only during pregnancy but also *during her entire life.*

Burke[5] correlated the nutritional value of the mother's diet with the early development of the newborn child. A pediatrician rated the physical condition of infants immediately after birth and throughout the following 2 weeks. Each mother's diet was evaluated as well. It was concluded that there was a significant relationship between the diet of the mother and the physical condition of the infant. It was further indicated that if the mother's diet during pregnancy is poor, her chances of having an infant in poor physical condition are increased. In a similar study, Dieckman[19] found that a pediatrician's assessment of several infants' physical condition correlated closely with the protein intake of the mother during pregnancy. Recently there has been emphasis on the possible long-term effects of maternal nutritional deprivation upon the physical and mental development of the infant. Although the data are as yet incomplete, they tend to indicate a much higher incidence of developmental abnormalities in protein-deficient infants and children.

It would appear from the research on maternal age that the most opportune time for conception of a healthy baby is between the ages of 20 and 30 years.[22] Haynes[29] indicated that when maternal age is under 16 years or over 36 years for the first born or over 40 years for additional children, the mother runs a greater risk of giving birth to a neurologically defective child.

Maternal age is of special significance in the chromosome disorder Down's syndrome, or mongolism, which occurs with greater frequency among infants born to older mothers. Mongolism affects approximately one in every 700.[7] A mother over the age of 45 has a 1-in-50 chance of giving birth to a child with Down's syndrome, whereas a mother of 25 would have a chance of only 1 in 2000.[28]

Many infectious agents are potentially harmful to the developing fetus. Maternal infections may harm the fetus by causing deformities during the early stages of fetal development, or they may be passed directly to the fetus and result in a congenital infection of the newborn infant. The most thoroughly studied maternal infection is the rubella virus. It has been estimated that approximately one of every ten women does not contract rubella (German measles) during childhood and therefore remains susceptible to the condition during a pregnancy.[39] The earlier an expectant mother contracts the virus during pregnancy, the greater her chance of producing a child with some birth defect (Table 2–1).

A woman infected with rubella during the first month of pregnancy has a 50 per cent chance of affecting her unborn child, whereas a woman who

Table 2–1 CONGENITAL DEFECTS RELATED TO RUBELLA*

GESTATIONAL AGE AT WHICH RUBELLA WAS CONTRACTED BY THE MOTHER (WEEKS)	RISK OF CONGENITAL DEFECTS (PER CENT)	PROBABLE TYPES OF DEFECTS
1–4	30–50	Cardiac lesions, eye lesions, glaucoma
4–8	25	Hearing defects
9–12	8	Psychomotor retardation
13–16	71	Primarily hearing defects

*Adapted from Clausen, Joy P., et al.: *Maternity Nursing Today*, p. 758. Copyright © by McGraw-Hill, Inc. Used with permission of McGraw-Hill Book Company.

contracts the virus during the second three months has only a 10 per cent risk of producing a child with some birth impairment. It has been estimated that some 20,000 to 30,000 children were handicapped as a result of the rubella epidemic of 1963–65. Approximately 10,000 of these children suffered mild to moderate impairments such as learning disabilities, educable mental retardation, or mild sensory disorders. The remaining children suffered severe sensory impairment or mental retardation.[6] The effects upon the developing fetus of other maternal infections such as measles, chicken pox, smallpox, and mumps are still under investigation.

Rh blood incompatibility may also adversely affect later motor development in young children. The Rh factor is a protein substance present on the red blood cells of approximately 85 per cent of all humans, while the remaining 15 per cent are Rh negative.[20] A difficulty arises when an Rh negative woman conceives with an Rh positive man and the resulting fetus is also Rh positive. During delivery of the first Rh positive baby, some of the baby's red blood cells containing antigens may infiltrate the mother's blood. The mother becomes sensitive to this positive blood and forms antibodies against the new Rh antigens in her blood. Since this takes place at birth, the first child is not affected. In subsequent positive pregnancies, however, this sensitivity may become more acute and may cause a jaundiced condition that could harm the fetus' neurological system or in severe cases cause death. An Rh negative mother can receive a Rho GAM injection within 72 hours of the termination of each Rh positive pregnancy, which limits the mother's production of antibodies against Rh positive blood and thereby reduces the risk of additional Rh positive pregnancies.[8]

The effect of drugs upon the fetus has been an area of concern to expectant mothers and the medical profession. The thalidomide tragedy of the early 1960's has alerted many individuals to the potential dangers of taking some drugs during pregnancy. Many commonly used drugs may be passed directly through the placenta to the fetus. As a precaution, doctors generally have their patients avoid the extensive use of drugs during pregnancy because little conclusive research concerning the effect of many drugs upon the embryo is available. It is generally accepted, however, that numerous drugs, including over-the-counter medications, may harm the developing infant if taken early in pregnancy. The use of addicting, narcotic drugs by an expectant mother increases the risk of prematurity, breech presentation, or premature rupture of the membranes. More than half of all narcotic-dependent babies weigh less than $5\frac{1}{2}$ pounds at birth.[36]

The effect of maternal smoking and alcoholism upon the developing fetus has been the subject of various studies. It may be concluded from the results of these studies that maternal smoking tends to reduce an infant's birth weight. Jones and Smith[32] found that children born to alcoholic mothers suffer from a "fetal alcoholic syndrome" and have a high incidence of pre- and postnatal growth deficiencies and developmental lags.

Radiation from excessive or careless use of x-rays during the early stages of pregnancy may also negatively influence the embryo's development. Therefore, x-rays should be used with utmost care on a pregnant patient and should be delayed, if possible, until after the pregnancy.

NATAL INFLUENCES

During the birth process, numerous factors may influence the child's later growth and development. At the onset of labor, the fetus begins a trying journey into an environment that is extremely different from the comfort and warmth of the mother's womb.

Abnormal contractions during labor may cause labor to be too rapid or too prolonged. Prolonged labor, which may be caused by uncoordinated or weak contractions of the uterus, subjects the infant to greater chances of anoxia and cerebral damage. Extremely strong contractions of the uterus may place excessive pressure upon the membranes of the skull, causing them to rupture, or the intense pressure may damage the infant's skull and lead to cerebral hemorrhage.[33]

The position of the fetus during labor is an important consideration in determining possible risks to the newborn. Approximately 4 per cent of all deliveries are breech presentations in which the infant passes through the birth canal in an inverted or buttocks-first position.[12] Injuries suffered during breech births include damage to the infant's brain and spinal cord. Many factors, including the size of the infant's head and the mother's pelvis, excessively forceful contractions, too rapid a delivery of the head, or the injurious use of forceps, contribute to these injuries.[44] After diagnosing the infant in a breech position, the obstetrician must decide whether to allow the mother to give birth normally or to perform a cesarean section.

During the birth process, the infant is supplied with oxygen from the placenta and umbilical cord. If the placenta separates from the uterine wall prematurely, or if the cord becomes knotted, compressed, or ruptures, the infant will be severed from its mother's oxygen supply and risk anoxia. The cord may also become tangled around the infant's neck or abdomen, cutting off the fetal blood supply.

Obstetricians, pediatricians, and parents commonly use birth weight as an indication of the health of the newborn. Infants born below normal weight are usually classified as "premature" or "full-term low–birth weight" babies. Approximately 300,000 of these infants are born each year. The premature infant is usually born after a short (under 36 weeks) intrauterine life. The infant of low birth weight, however, is born near full term but has experienced some intrauterine developmental retardation.

Prematurity is a major cause of infant mortality in the United States. The infants who survive tend to exhibit a greater incidence of neurological damage than children of normal birth weight.[20] Shirley[41] studied children identified as immature at birth during their first 2 years of life. She showed that the premature infant is physiologically underdeveloped at birth and thereby subject to a greater chance of cerebral and neurological injury at birth. Because the bone structure of the premature infant is not fully developed, the skull is subject to a greater chance of injury during the birth process.[8] After 2 years of observing and testing each child, she concluded that ". . . prematurity manifests itself more definitely in motor than non-motor development."

The premature infant has less chance of a developmental lag than does the infant who is born under birth weight at full term. Babson et al.[2] observed that children born near full term who were classified as underdeveloped by this study failed to match the later physical and mental development of children of comparable birth weight born prematurely.

The retarded development that begins while infants of very low birth weight are still in the uterus appears to continue during the child's later growth and development. Between 1940 and 1960 Drillien[21] studied a total of 97 infants with birth weights of 3 pounds or less. Forty-nine of the children had passed their fifth birthday at the time of the study. The results indicated that half of these students were uneducable in normal schools because of physical and mental impairments. One-quarter of the children were classified as dull, requiring special education services, while the remaining students were classified as low average, average, or superior in educational ability.

POSTNATAL DETERMINANTS

From the moment of birth the infant's developmental potential will be affected by numerous factors. Those postnatal determinants that directly influence a child's motor development include: (1) the rate of physical and neurological maturation; (2) the quality and variety of the child's movement experiences; and (3) the conditions, either environmentally or genetically caused, that may affect motor efficiency.

The degree to which maturation and experience each influence motor development has been continually questioned. There have been several studies that utilize identical twins to determine the respective roles of maturation and experience in motor development.

Gesell and Thompson[26] conducted a study to discover the effect of special training upon the locomotor and manipulative behavior of identical twins. They concluded that learning these behaviors was dependent primarily on maturation, although experience is a factor in skill acquisition.

In a study of children 1 to 4 years of age who lived in Iranian institutions, Dennis[16] demonstrated the effects of environmental deprivation upon behavior development of these children. In two of the institutions the behavior development of the infants was greatly retarded, while the children in the third institution exhibited more normal behavior. The procedures of all three institutions were compared, and it was concluded that the retarded development of the children in the first two institutions may have been due to restrictions resulting from specific kinds of learning experiences. Children whose experience was limited not only had retarded motor development but also in many cases never developed certain patterns of motor development. Dennis concluded that experience affects both the time at which a motor skill appears and the very form of the skill.[16]

Singer[42] noted that some students have difficulty learning motor skills because of a lack of experience with movement patterns during childhood. He contended that learning a new motor skill depends upon prior movement experiences and that the basic movements acquired during early childhood form the basis of all later sport skills. Although they believed that many movement patterns are innate, Cooper and Glassow[10] indicated that these patterns improve with practice and that if not practiced at the time when they appear naturally, they may never develop into skills. Halverson[27] stated that, although it is true that many children may attain a rudimentary level of fundamental movement patterns, they may never master the mature form of the movement.

Both maturation and experience play important roles in the development of fundamental movement patterns during early childhood. Initial motor patterns tend to be maturationally based, while the refinement of those movements is dependent upon past movement experiences. With increasing age and more complex motor development, the *quality* and *variety* of a child's movement experiences figure significantly in the development of mature movement patterns. Although all children achieve an initial or rudimentary level of functioning, these patterns are refined only through continual practice and exploration.

Although many children develop inefficient fundamental movement patterns because of a lack of proper basic movement experiences during early childhood, there are other postnatal factors that may influence a child's movement abilities. Injuries to the brain, infections that affect the central nervous system, tumors, and some poisons, in addition to the numerous prenatal and natal influences previously noted, may cause neurological impairment, which may be exhibited in varying degrees, depending upon the child's condition.

In recent years there has been a keen interest in the child who functions normally in the academic setting but demonstrates poorly coordinated movements when performing motor patterns. Arnheim and Sinclair[1] identified these children as victims of the *"clumsy child syndrome."* These children of low motor ability are found in all school settings; Cratty[11] indicated that approximately 8 to 10 per cent of normal school populations show some form of minimal to moderate neurological dysfunction.

In addition to low-normal motor function, there are various other conditions that may affect a child's ability to perform fundamental movement patterns efficiently. Cruickshank and Johnson[14] defined the exceptional child as "one who deviates intellectually, physically, socially, and emotionally so much from what is considered to be normal growth and development that he cannot receive maximum benefit from a regular school program and requires a special class of supplementary instruction and services." Many times the exact cause of a motor impairment is difficult to identify because of the numerous exceptional characteristics that a child may manifest. The redundance of terminology dealing with the exceptional child compounds the difficulty. This lack of common terms, as well as the abusive use of flowery labels, was demonstrated by Fry[24] in his terminology generator (Table 2–2).

It has been estimated that about 12 per cent or 7 million, of American school age children are emotionally, physically, or mentally handicapped. Approximately 45 per cent of these children are not being offered special educational services.[34] With the current emphasis upon putting exceptional

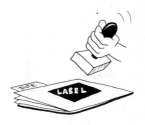

Table 2-2 DO-IT-YOURSELF TERMINOLOGY GENERATOR

Directions: Select any word from Column 1. Add any word from Column 2, then add any word from Column 3. If you don't like the result, try again. It will mean about the same thing.

QUALIFIER	AREA OF INVOLVEMENT	PROBLEM
Minimal	Brain	Dysfunction
Mild	Cerebral	Damage
Minor	Neurologic	Disorder
Chronic	Neurological	Dissynchronization
Diffuse	Central Nervous System	Handicap
Specific	Language	Disability
Primary	Reading	Retardation
Disorganized	Perceptual	Impairment
Organic	Impulse	Pathology
Clumsy	Behavior	Syndrome

The above system will yield 1000 terms.

Adapted from Fry, Edward: Do-it-yourself terminology generator. *Journal of Reading, 11*:428, 1968. Used with permission.

children into the mainstream of education and upon new legislation to support the process, state departments of education are required to provide educational services to all children without regard to their limitations.

Public Law 94–142 requires school districts to provide all handicapped children with a free, appropriate public education, including special education and other related services. This act further stipulates that physical education should be included as a component of special education services of the handicapped. Physical education is further defined as "...special physical education, adapted physical education and motor development; [physical education] means the development of physical and motor fitness, fundamental motor skills and patterns..."* To comply with this ruling, school districts will need additional specially trained physical educators or will require supplementary training for present members of their staffs.

Current research indicates that handicapped children exhibit a greater

*Federal Register, Vol. 41, No. 252, Washington, D.C.: U.S. Department of Health, Education, and Welfare, Dec. 30, 1976, p. 56978.

percentage of motor impairments than do normal children. Numerous studies have shown that mentally retarded children fail to keep pace with normal children in their motor development.[23, 30, 31, 47] Similar results have been found with children classified as "minimally brain injured."[3] Children with sensory handicaps also tend to exhibit a lag in motor development.[4, 45] At this time, however, it is difficult to determine whether the motor deficiency experienced by children with sensory impairments results from organic disorders or from limited opportunities for movement during early development.

SUMMARY

This chapter has dealt with general aspects of motor development during early childhood and the role of fundamental movement patterns in later skill development. In addition, the major prenatal, natal and postnatal influences on motor development were discussed.

Children develop movement skills in a progressively more complex manner, from early involuntary reflexive movements to highly complex skills. The period of early childhood (2 to 7 years of age) appears to be critical in the development of fundamental movement patterns. Children who do not develop mature movement patterns during this period later often have difficulty performing more complex sport skills.

Movement patterns develop in a series of identifiable stages. As each pattern passes through the initial, elementary, and mature stages, distinct, observable changes take place in body actions. Although most children will develop the initial form of a movement pattern regardless of external influences, children need appropriate movement experiences to refine each pattern into an efficient, mature form.

It is clear that children begin developing fundamental movement patterns prior to reaching school age, and the first few years at school are spent molding these patterns into highly coordinated movements. It is the duty of parents and preschool and elementary school teachers to give their children opportunities for numerous movement experiences.

Children should be given freedom to explore various movement activities, and fathers should spend time playing ball with their daughters as well as their sons. Children who have experienced some prenatal or natal complication should especially be offered opportunities to participate in physical activity successfully.

Elementary classroom teachers without the advantage of assistance from a trained physical education specialist should provide their students not with a "free play period" but rather with a planned program of movement experience geared to building and perfecting fundamental patterns of movement. Teachers should be knowledgeable about the progressive development of fundamental movement patterns during early childhood, and they should be able to identify students in their classes who are behind in their motor development.

Elementary physical educators should design curricula that take into account the development of motor skills. The early elementary years should be spent in mastering fundamental patterns, and during the later elementary years these patterns should be utilized in developing basic sport-related skills. Teachers should establish programs to aid the motor development of students having difficulty with fundamental patterns.

Throughout the developmental process, many factors may adversely affect a child's motor development. Children who possess exceptional characteristics should receive special attention in the physical education program. Special educators and physical educators who conduct special physical education classes, as well as regular physical education teachers, should be particularly aware of children who are having trouble performing mature movement patterns. Early physical education experiences should be designed to develop fundamental movement patterns through physical activities appropriate for the age of the students.

BIBLIOGRAPHY

1. Arnheim, Daniel, and Sinclair, William: *The Clumsy Child.* St. Louis: C. V. Mosby Co., 1975, 231 pp.
2. Babson, Gorham, et al.: Growth and development of twins of dissimilar size at birth. *Pediatrics, 33*:327–33, 1964.
3. Boardhead, Geoffrey: Gross motor performance in minimally brain injured children. *Journal of Motor Behavior, 4*:103–10, 1972.
4. Buell, Charles: Motor performance of visually-handicapped children. *Journal of Exceptional Children, 17*:69–72, 1950.
5. Burke, Bertha S., et al.: Influence of nutrition during pregnancy upon the condition of the infant at birth. *Journal of Nutrition, 26*:569–83, 1943.
6. Calvert, Donald R.: Report on Rubella and Handicapped Children. Washington, D.C.: Bureau of Education for the Handicapped, U.S. Department of Health, Education, and Welfare, May 1967, 7 pp.
7. Chromosome 21 and Its Association with Down's Syndrome. White Plains, N.Y.: The National Foundation of the March of Dimes.
8. Clausen, Joy P., et al.: *Maternity Nursing Today.* New York: McGraw-Hill, 1973.
9. Committee on Maternal Nutrition: Maternal Nutrition and the Course of Pregnancy. Washington, D.C.: National Academy of Science, 1970, 241 pp.
10. Cooper, John M., and Glassow, Ruth B.: *Kinesiology.* St. Louis: C. V. Mosby Co., 1972, 332 pp.
11. Cratty, Bryant J.: *Remedial Motor Activity for Children.* Philadelphia: Lea and Febiger, 1975, 327 pp.
12. Crawley, Lawrence, et al.: *Reproduction, Sex, and Preparation for Marriage,* 2nd ed. Englewood Cliffs, N.J.: Prentice-Hall, 1973, 254 pp.
13. Cruickshank, William M.: *The Brain Injured Child in Home, School, and Community.* Syracuse, N.Y.: Syracuse University Press, 1967, 294 pp.
14. Cruickshank, William M., and Johnson, Orville G.: *Education of Exceptional Children and Youth.* Englewood Cliffs, N.J.: Prentice-Hall, 1975, 780 pp.
15. Deach, Dorothy F.: Genetic Development of Motor Skills in Children Two Through Six Years of Age. Unpublished doctoral dissertation, University of Michigan, 1951, 401 pp.
16. Dennis, Wayne: Causes of retardation among institutional children: Iran. *Journal of Genetic Psychology, 96*:47–59, 1960.
17. Dennis, Wayne: Does culture appreciably affect patterns of infant behavior? *Journal of Social Psychology, 12*:305–17, 1940.
18. Dennis, Wayne: The effects of restricted practice upon the reaching, sitting, and standing of two infants. *Journal of Genetic Psychology, 47*:17–32, 1935.
19. Dieckman, W. J., et al.: Observations on protein intake and the health of the mother and baby: I. clinical and laboratory findings. *American Dietetic Association Journal, 27*: 1046–52, 1951.

20. Dileo, Joseph: *Physical Factors in Growth and Development.* New York: Teachers College Press, Columbia University, 1970, 58 pp.
21. Drillien, Cecil March: The incidence of mental and physical handicaps in school age children of very low birth weight. *Pediatrics, 21:*452–64, 1961.
22. Flowers, Charles E.: Prevention of Obstetric Accidents. Washington, D.C.: Proceedings of the National Conference for the Prevention of Mental Retardation Through Improved Maternity Care, March 27–29, 1968.
23. Francis, Robert J., and Rarick, G. Lawrence: Motor characteristics of the mentally retarded. *American Journal of Mental Deficiency, 63:*792–811, 1959.
24. Fry, Edward: Do-it-yourself terminology generator. *Journal of Reading, 11:*428, 1968.
25. Gallahue, David, Werner, Peter, and Luedke, George: *A Conceptual Approach to Moving and Learning.* New York: John Wiley, 1975, 423 pp.
26. Gesell, Arnold, and Thompson, Helen: *Infant Behavior: Its Genesis and Growth.* New York: McGraw-Hill, 1934, 343 pp.
27. Halverson, Lolas E.: Development of motor patterns in young children. *Quest VI, A Symposium on Motor Learning, 6:*44–53, 1966.
28. Happy Birthday from the Foundation. White Plains, N.Y.: The National Foundation of the March of Dimes.
29. Haynes, Una: A Developmental Approach to Case Finding. Washington, D.C.: Social Rehabilitation Services, U.S. Department of Health, Education, and Welfare, 1967, 85 pp.
30. Hollingsworth, Jack Darel: A Comparison of Motor Ability of Mentally Retarded Children of Specific Mental and Chronological Ages and Normal Children. Unpublished doctoral dissertation, University of Georgia, 1971, 80 pp.
31. Howe, Clifford E.: A comparison of motor skills of mentally retarded and normal children. *Exceptional Children, 25:*352–54, 1959.
32. Jones, Kenneth, and Smith, David W.: Recognition of the fetal alcohol syndrome in early infancy. *Lancet 2:*999–1001, 1973.
33. Lerch, Constance: *Maternity Nursing.* St. Louis: C. V. Mosby Co., 1974, 432 pp.
34. Mainstreaming, what it's all about. *Today's Education, 65:*18–19, 1976.
35. McGraw, Myrtle B.: *Growth: A Study of Johnny and Jimmy.* New York: Appleton-Century, 1935, 319 pp.
36. Neonatal Narcotic Dependence. Chevy Chase, Md.: National Clearinghouse for Drug Abuse Information, Report Series No. 29, 1974, 13 pp.
37. Perinatal Care. *Leader Alert Bulletin.* White Plains, N.Y.: The National Foundation of the March of Dimes.
38. Prenatal care to prevent birth defects. *Leader Alert Bulletin.* White Plains, N.Y.: The National Foundation of the March of Dimes, 1972.
39. Preventing birth defects caused by rubella and Rh blood disease. *Leader Alert Bulletin.* White Plains, N.Y.: The National Foundation of the March of Dimes.
40. Progress in prevention of birth defects, *Leader Alert Bulletin.* White Plains, N.Y.: The National Foundation of the March of Dimes.
41. Shirley, Mary: Development of immature babies during their first two years. *Child Development, 9:*347–60, 1938.
42. Singer, Robert N.: *Motor Learning and Human Performance.* New York: Macmillan, 1969, 354 pp.
43. Smith, Betty J.: The Reasons Women Receive or Do Not Receive Prenatal Care and the Reasons They Receive Early or Late Prenatal Care. Unpublished doctoral dissertation, Columbia University, 1971, 323 pp.
44. Tank, Edward S., et al.: Mechanisms of trauma during breech delivery. *Obstetrics and Gynecology, 38:*761, 1971.
45. Vance, Paul C.: Motor Characteristics of Deaf Children. Unpublished doctoral dissertation, University of Northern Colorado, 1968, 108 pp.
46. West, Max: *Prenatal Care.* Washington, D.C.: Children's Bureau, U.S. Department of Labor, 1924, 41 pp.
47. Widdop, James H.: The Motor Performance of Educable Mentally Retarded Children with Particular Reference to the Identification of Factors Associated with Individual Differences in Performance. Unpublished doctoral dissertation, University of Wisconsin, 1967, 242 pp.

CHAPTER 3

ACQUISITION OF FUNDAMENTAL LOCOMOTOR PATTERNS DURING EARLY CHILDHOOD

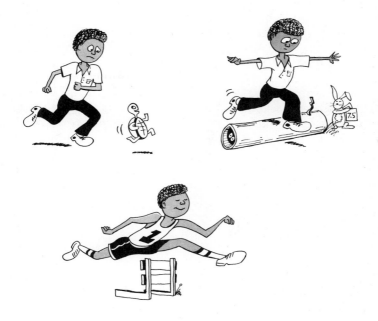

The Walking Pattern
The Running Pattern
The Jumping Pattern
Summary

Locomotor movements are exhibited early in an infant's development. The newborn may be stimulated to perform numerous involuntary reflexes that resemble later voluntary locomotor patterns. These early reflexes are gradually inhibited as the infant develops voluntary control over rudimentary forms of locomotion. The first attempts at purposeful locomotion involve an isolated pulling action of the arms in a creeping pattern. However, the infant slowly begins to synchronize the actions of the arms and legs in an efficient crawling pattern.

As the young child's strength and stability improve, he spends more time in supported upright postures. The first attempts at independent walking involve moving from one handhold to another. The initial attempts at stepping away from the handhold are at first unsuccessful, and the child often reverts to a more familiar and stable crawling pattern. The age at which independent walking begins is highly variable and may normally occur as early as the ninth month of life or as late as the eighteenth month, depending upon both the individual's experiences and level of maturation.

By about 24 months of age, most children have acquired an adequate walking pattern and thus begin to experiment with rudimentary forms of running. This point marks the end of infancy and the onset of early childhood. The child then begins a period in which he or she explores a variety of more complex fundamental movement patterns. During this time, individual body actions are continually being refined and integrated into more sophisticated patterns requiring increased strength and stability.

This chapter reviews the development of the fundamental locomotor patterns of walking, running, and the standing long jump. Current research on the acquisition of the locomotor patterns of hopping, skipping, and galloping is insufficient to allow the formation of definitive conclusions about their development and refinement during the early childhood period. Although acquired previous to the beginning of early childhood, the walking pattern does not mature until the child is approximately 3 years of age; therefore, a discussion of the walking pattern is included in this chapter.

THE WALKING PATTERN

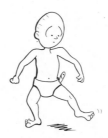

In acquiring the walking pattern, the infant progresses from a four-limbed locomotor pattern to a more efficient, upright biped pattern. Broer[3] defines the act of walking as ". . . a matter of disturbing the mechanical equilibrium of the body, by pushing the body forward, and forming successive new bases by moving the legs forward alternately."

The walking pattern passes through a series of increasingly complex stages, beginning with the first uncoordinated and unstable steps and ending with a highly integrated and refined movement. Before an infant is able to attempt independent walking successfully, he needs to develop sufficient leg strength to support his body weight and propel it forward and adequate stability to maintain equilibrium in an upright posture.[10] A child usually develops these necessary skills between the ages of 9 and 18 months, and thereafter spends increasing amounts of time in exploring the walking pattern unsupported. Several studies have focused on the various stages in the infant's acquisition of an independent gait pattern.

Shirley[18] extensively investigated the development of 25 children during the first 2 years of life and identified four stages in the acquisition of the walking pattern. The children who were observed initially exhibited a dancing, or patting and stepping, motion when held in a supported position. The infants were gradually able to stand with support, bearing most of the weight on their feet while attempting to maintain balance with their arms. With maturation the infants could vary the size of the stepping angle and finally developed the skills needed to walk unsupported successfully. During the final stage, the speed of the walk rapidly increased as the stride lengthened, the base of support narrowed, and the angle of the step decreased.

McGraw[16] observed 82 children ranging in age from a few months to 8 years. She identified seven phases in the development of a mature walking pattern (Table 3–1).

In a study designed to determine when various gait characteristics appear after independent locomotion begins, Burnett and Johnson[4] filmed 28 children (13 males, 15 females) at approximately 4-week intervals at or before the onset of independent walking. Eighteen of the children studied had not yet achieved an independent gait, although all could bear their weight with support. These prewalkers gradually developed the stability and coordination skills necessary for a successful walking pattern. Initial attempts at stepping were characterized by little flexion of the hip and lower extremities, and trunk rotation moved the lead leg forward. An early pelvic tilt, observed in several prewalkers, was attributed to uncoordination because of its frequent disappearance during the first weeks of walking.

Burnett and Johnson also observed that initial attempts at walking were characterized by a wide base of support to compensate for immature stability skills. The lower extremities were externally rotated and abducted throughout the swing. As the walking pattern matured, the legs swung in a controlled manner and the base of support narrowed. The children developed a heel strike, a flexion at midstance, and a mature foot and knee action by the fifty-fifth week after they had achieved an independent gait. Similarly, the arms were initially held in an abducted, externally rotated, and flexed position and later began to swing in synchronized opposition to the legs.

In studying infants' coordination of locomotion, Burnside[5] concluded that they progress from pulling the body with the arms only to moving by using both the arms and the legs and finally to attainment of an upright posture and an independent gait. She emphasized the importance of stability in

Table 3–1   McGRAW'S PHASES OF ACQUISITION OF THE WALKING PATTERN

PHASE	CHARACTERISTICS
Newborn or reflexive stepping	When held upright, the infant assumes a position of general flexion. Some of the observed infants exhibited localized stepping movements that became somewhat more prevalent during the first 3 weeks.
Inhibition or static	The infant progressively inhibits the reflexive stepping movements and gains increasing postural control. The head is held steady, and there is less flexion in the upper and lower extremities.
Transition	The infant shows greater body activity and tends to move his body in an up and down fashion while holding his feet stationary, or he may stand and stamp his feet or make a stepping motion.
Deliberate stepping	The infant's stepping motions and postural control become more deliberate, but cortical control of posture and stepping has not yet been integrated. The child must still be given support, although the amount of aid needed decreases.
Independent stepping	The infant has developed sufficient stability, strength, and coordination to engage in independent walking. The arms are extended and abducted, with the fingers extended as well. The feet are positioned wide apart for increased stability, and there is marked flexion at the knees and hips. The steps are high and isolated, and the toes grip the floor for balance.
Heel-toe progression	Coordination improves as the infant begins to walk in a heel-toe progression in which the heel of the front foot hits the ground as the toes of the rear foot are lifted. The arms are held to the side with the fingers relaxed, as the base of support narrows and the legs swing in a more controlled manner.
Integration, or maturity of erect locomotion	The infant's arms swing in a synchronized action in opposition to the lower extremities. Initially, the arms swing from the forearms, and with maturity the arms swing in a regular rhythmical manner from the shoulders.

Adapted from McGraw, Myrtle: *The Neuromuscular Maturation of the Human Infant.* New York: Columbia University Press, 1943. Used with permission.

the refinement of the walking pattern. The young child's high center of gravity, small base of support, low body weight, and poor coordination of the muscles required to maintain balance all contribute to poor stability. She observed that children compensate for these factors by widening their base of support, flexing at the hip and knee to lower the center of gravity, and raising the arms to aid in coordination. As the pattern becomes more refined, the length of the step increases, the base of support narrows, and the stepping action becomes more regular. Burnside further noted that with development the arms flex at the elbows with the forearms held forward and then hang easily at the sides.

Cratty[8] found that a child's first attempts to walk are characterized by a wide base of support, a toeing-out of the feet, and an irregular rhythmical gait (Fig. 3–1). The walking pattern becomes more rhythmical as the width of the step gradually decreases and the stepping angle straightens. He further noted that initially an infant must visually attend to his feet, whereas the older child can walk without having to monitor his steps visually.

Godfrey and Kephart[14] observed that many children have difficulty in directing the sequence of the walking pattern even though they are able to perform all the actions that constitute the movement. Because young children also have trouble flexing the lower extremities, the movement appears jerky, stiff, and jarring.

As walking develops and stability improves, children are able to perform a more complicated walking pattern; they gain greater proficiency in their ability to stop, start, and turn while walking. In a study conducted by Wellman,[20] children 37 months of age were able to walk a distance of 10 feet along a straight line without stepping off, whereas it was not until 8 months later that they could successfully walk a circular path.

Because walking begins prior to early childhood and because most children at 2 years of age have developed a fairly refined walking pattern, the pattern will not be described in relation to the three developmental stages of early childhood but rather in terms of general developmental trends.

The walking pattern passes through a series of stages that require increasing strength, stability, and coordination skills. Initial attempts at locomotion involve a creeping pattern in which the infant uses his arms to propel himself. Gradually the infant pulls his legs under his hips and uses them in a more efficient crawling motion. When held upright, the young infant exhibits a general flexion throughout the limbs and often performs a rapid, unrhythmical, stepping motion. As the motor system matures and as strength and stability improve, the infant is able to support increasing amounts of body weight on his feet. The infant often makes awkward stepping motions until he is finally able to walk when supported with both hands. With further development the infant is gradually able to step away successfully from the support and walk independently.

To summarize, the initial walking pattern is unstable and uncoordinated; thus the infant often falls. Throughout the remaining 3 years of early childhood, this locomotor pattern becomes highly refined and integrated. A wide base of support, a toeing-out of the feet, and an unrhythmical stepping

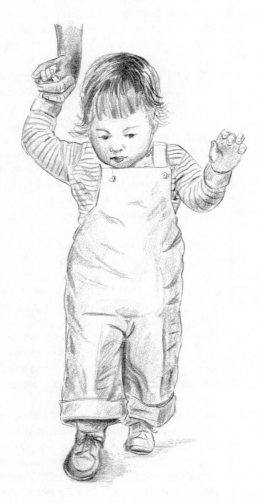

Figure 3–1 Front view of early walking pattern. Note the outward rotation of the swinging leg as the arms are held abducted and flexed at the elbow.

action are distinctive features of early attempts at walking. In addition, the arms are held high, away from the sides, and slightly flexed for balance and protection in case of a fall. As the walking pattern is refined, the base of support narrows and the length and speed of the step increase. Walking becomes rhythmical as the heel of the foot makes contact with the ground. The legs swing in a controlled manner, and the stepping angle decreases. The arms are held at the side and swing from the shoulder in synchronized opposition to the legs.

THE RUNNING PATTERN

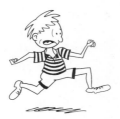

As a child's walking pattern becomes more secure, he begins to explore various other forms of locomotion for moving more efficiently in his environment. A child's normal play activities involve numerous opportunities for running. As these play experiences become organized into games, sport, and recreational activities, running becomes essential for successful participation.

The actions of the upper and lower extremities in running are similar to those exhibited in walking. Running at first tends to resemble a fast walk because there is no observable flight phase in which the child is totally unsupported. The initial running pattern is characterized by unstable and uncoordinated movements. By approximately 18 months of age, the child has developed the stability necessary for successful walking. As the speed of the walk increases, the child finds it more difficult to maintain balance. To compensate, the child often reverts to using features of immature walking, such as a wide base of support and an abducted arm position.

Rarick[17] observed that the initial running pattern is characterized by stiff movements, uneven strides, and a jarring gait but that with development the stride evens and running becomes smoother. Sinclair[19] noted that as stability skills become greater and as stride length is increased, the base of support is narrowed and the support phase is shortened. Contact with the ground is made closer to the ball of the foot as the child leans forward for a faster start.

Several studies have identified developmental trends in the acquisition of a skillful running pattern and the changes in body actions that result in pattern refinements. Glassow, Halverson, and Rarick[13] reported that with development, the stride increases, the contact time is shortened, and the percentage of time in flight increases from grade one to grade six. They also observed that as the foot reaches the ground at the end of the flight, the contact point changes from the heel to the ball of the foot; the knee of the swinging leg flexes more, and the thigh of that leg more nearly approaches the perpendicular.

Using film, Clouse[6] studied the running patterns of six boys ranging in age from 14 to 59 months for a period of 8 months. Analysis of the films revealed several developmental trends in the acquisition of a skillful running pattern (Fig. 3–2). She observed that as the boys got older, they spent more time in the flight phase of the pattern, their running speed and stride length increased, and the vertical distance moved by the center of gravity decreased in relation to the horizontal distance of the stride. The support leg was extended more forcefully, and the older subjects utilized leg extension more effectively than the younger runners, who were likely to start flexion before takeoff. The recovery thigh tended with age to be swung faster and through a larger range.

She summarized the conclusions of her study:

1. Changes in the running pattern occur during the preschool years, and they can be identified and measured.

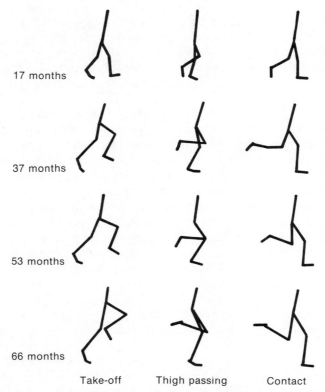

17 months

37 months

53 months

66 months

Take-off   Thigh passing   Contact

Figure 3–2 Progressive development of the leg action of the running pattern. (Adapted from Clouse, Florence Cuthill: A Kinematic Analysis of the Development of the Running Pattern of Preschool Boys. Unpublished doctoral dissertation, University of Wisconsin, 1959.)

2. Measurement of these changes reveals definite developmental trends in the age range observed.
3. Developmental trends in running can be logically related to improved mechanics of running and, therefore, represent progress toward a skillful pattern.

Dittmer[9] attempted to identify the mechanics of the running pattern of grade school girls and to isolate factors that resulted in good or poor performance. Four subjects 6 years of age were studied for 4 years. Two subjects were rated as good performers and two as poor performers on the basis of their scores for running a distance of 30 yards. The results of this study were divided into two parts.

Conclusions about the presence of developmental trends in the subjects' patterns were drawn first. From the results of her longitudinal study, Dittmer noted that with each additional year of age, there was an increase in the length and speed of each performer's stride. She further concluded that with maturity there was more noncontact, or time when there is no supporting limb in contact with the ground. Moreover, the portion of contact time used for propulsion increased, while the amount of contact time spent on recovery decreased. With further development, the knee flexed progressively more during the recovery, during the forward swing of the leg, and at landing.

Dittmer also studied characteristic differences in the running patterns of the good and poor performers. She concluded that good runners, with age, exhibited a longer and faster stride, a lower percentage of contact time, and a greater flexibility of the lower extremities than poorer performers. Better performers also tended to land with more of their weight over the support foot and had a lower angle at takeoff, thus throwing their weight farther beyond the support foot.

Fortney[12] conducted a longitudinal study of the swinging limb of 12 boys 7 through 11 years of age. Over a period of 5 years, she found changes in both good and poor performers. She discovered that with an increase in age, the leading thigh tended to be lifted higher at the beginning of the nonsupport phase. During the support phase, there was a progressive flexion of the recovery knee that brought the foot closer to the buttocks as it began its forward swing. Children rated as good performers exhibited a higher heel kick as the thigh was swung forward faster and higher through a larger arc.

In an early study, Anderson and Randall[1] discovered some factors that influence speed in running. They concluded that there is a close correlation between speed and the angle of the knee of the push-off leg. They observed that faster runners have a higher recovery kick and bring their leg forward in a more flexed position, and in a higher plane, than do slower runners. Faster runners also had a longer stride than slower runners. Finally, the angle of the body (body lean) was not found to be a highly significant factor in the speed of running.

Beck[2] studied the movement of the center of gravity during running in terms of distance, time, and velocity in order to determine its path through space and to show the grade level at which changes in performance occurred. Twelve boys were divided into three subgroups with four boys in each. During the first year of the study, the children were in grades one, three, and five; the following year they advanced one grade, giving a sample of all six grades. Beck concluded that the path of the center of gravity during running is wavelike in appearance and similar for all subjects regardless of age.

Beck further noted that with an increase in age, the center of gravity moved farther horizontally than vertically. Since there is more progress made in the horizontal plane, the run becomes smoother as the child gets older. The study also corroborates other research that indicates that as the running pattern develops, support receives less time than flight and propulsion receives greater time than recovery.

Although there is limited information regarding the rear view of the legs and the action of the arms during the running pattern, Wickstrom[21] reported some tentative observations. He found that a young child, when running at full speed, swings the recovery knee outward, then around and forward to the support position. In addition to this knee swing, there is a tendency for the young child to toe-out the swinging foot, which allows the foot to swing forward without being raised more than a few inches. This outward knee swing, Wickstrom contended, later produces the pattern in which the recovery foot first crosses over the child's midline toward the rear before it swings around and forward (Fig. 3–3). The rotary leg actions seem to disappear with development. "A regular increase in the length of the running stride contributes significantly to the elimination of the less productive rotary leg movements."

The arms are an integral component of the running pattern. Wickstrom[21] has recognized several trends in the development of mature arm action. During the first stages of running, the legs are stiff and the strides are

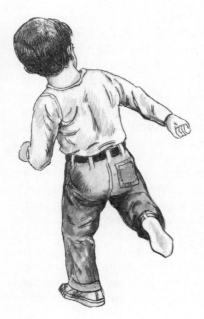

Figure 3–3 Rear view of elementary running pattern. Note the excessive rotation of the recovery leg on the forward swing. This causes the arms to swing outward to maintain stability.

short. There is very little bend in the arms, and the arcs in which the arms swing are short. As the child rotates his recovery knee, the opposite arm makes a hooking motion forward toward the midline of the body. As development progresses, the arms loop outward less on the backswing, pass through a longer arc in the anteroposterior plane, and are bent at the elbows in approximate right angles.

To summarize, the running pattern in early childhood is refined from an uncoordinated, unstable movement to a highly integrated and efficient pattern. During the developmental process, observable changes take place in the running pattern as the child acquires the ability to integrate complex body actions into a coordinated movement: the stride evens and lengthens as the percentage of time spent on the flight phase increases; the pattern becomes smoother as the legs absorb the shock of striking the ground; the trailing foot is recovered higher toward the rear before it is swung forward faster and higher; the arms are utilized more effectively as they swing in opposition to the legs; and as stability develops, the child is able to increase the degree of forward body lean during the initial strides of the run (Fig. 3–4 A and B).

During the early childhood period, the running pattern passes through three stages of development—initial, elementary, and mature. Each successive stage requires increases in strength, coordination, and stability as the

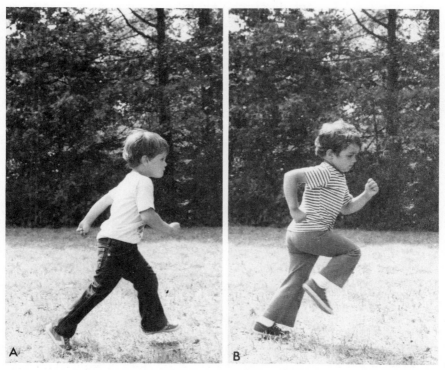

Figure 3–4 Observable differences in the running pattern of two children. Note the differences in arm and leg action.

pattern is refined and performance improves. The development of the running pattern may be summarized as follows.

The initial stage of the running pattern is characterized by a stiff and uneven stride with the base of support widened for increased stability. The recovery leg is limited in its swing and tends to exhibit an exaggerated outward rotation during the forward swing to a position of support. The foot toes outward as it strikes the ground flatfootedly. The extension of the support leg is incomplete, and there is no observable flight phase to the pattern since the child remains in contact with the running surface. The arms, held stiff with little flexion at the elbow, tend to be abducted to aid in maintaining equilibrium.

The elementary stage of the running pattern may be identified by an increased stride length as the run becomes faster. The recovery leg swings through a larger arc with a slight outward rotation. The foot strikes the ground straighter and closer to the toes. Prior to a short flight phase, the support leg extends more completely. The arms swing mainly from the elbows in opposition to the legs.

During the mature stage, the recovery leg is increasingly flexed and the foot is brought close to the buttocks as it begins its forward swing. The thigh of the swinging leg is quickly brought forward and high through a larger arc. The support leg extends completely through the hip, knee, and ankle. The flight phase is obvious, and the support leg bends slightly at contact to absorb the shock of landing. Less time is spent in the support position, and a greater percentage of the time is utilized for propulsion than for recovery. The arms move in a large arc from the shoulders and are bent at the elbows in approximate right angles.

THE JUMPING PATTERN

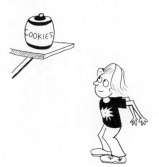

Jumping is a locomotor pattern in which the extension of the leg propels the body through space. The jumping pattern may be divided into four distinct phases: the preparatory crouch, takeoff, flight, and landing. Rarick[17] observed that the jump is a complicated modification of the previously established walking and running patterns. The jumping pattern requires the infant to further develop both leg strength to propel the body into flight and stability to maintain balance during the jumping action.

The sequential acquisition of jumping ability has been studied by numerous authors. Hillebrandt et al.[15] noted that children exhibit jumping patterns long before they are strong enough to propel their bodies into flight. An infant's initial experiences with jumping usually involve an exaggerated step down from a low height. This pattern requires a minimal amount of leg strength because of its downward motion with gravity rather than against it. The infant also compensates for his lack of stability skills by remaining in contact with the jumping surface; the stepping motion of the feet allows the lead foot to land before the infant lifts the rear support foot.

As his leg strength and stability improve, the child is able to jump from progressively greater heights and begin to propel himself into flight. Gradually the legs become sufficiently strong and stable both to propel the child into space and to land simultaneously. Hillebrandt et al.[15] indicated that in young children the leg action of the jumping pattern is far more advanced than the arm action. During the initial stages of development, the arms are held almost immobile. With maturation the arms are utilized for stability, and gradually they augment the action of the legs and thus add to the momentum of the jump. As the infant is able to integrate his arm action with his increasing leg strength and stability, height or distance in performance will rapidly improve (Fig. 3–5).

Although the ability to jump may actually be innate, it appears that the use of that ability in a more complex pattern, such as the standing long jump and the vertical jump, comes only through practice.[10] These jumps traditionally have been utilized to evaluate a child's leg power and jumping skill.

Wickstrom[21] noted that a developmental change takes place in the standing broad jump as the direction of thrust moves from the vertical toward the horizontal plane, thereby leading to a more mature pattern. As the ability to do the standing broad jump improves, there is a more definite preliminary crouch and the arms swing increasingly forward in the anteroposterior plane. During the takeoff there is a more complete extension of the body while there is a decrease in the angle of takeoff. The hip flexes more during flight, and the angle of the leg at landing decreases.

In a study investigating the kinesiological characteristics of good and poor performers in the standing broad jump, Felton[11] discovered that the velocity of the center of gravity was much greater for good jumpers than for poor jumpers. Good jumpers had greater flexion in all joints, which provided these jumpers with a greater distance through which to extend their bodies. Another conclusion drawn from this study was that good jumpers had more extension in the hip, knee, and ankle than poor jumpers. Felton also noted that good jumpers achieved a greater reach upon landing.

Glassow, Halverson, and Rarick[13] determined that although changes in the takeoff position are small with respect to age, the thigh and the trunk do move closer to the horizontal plane. Moreover, the time in flight increases, and upon landing, the thigh and the trunk move closer to the horizontal and the leg moves closer to the perpendicular.

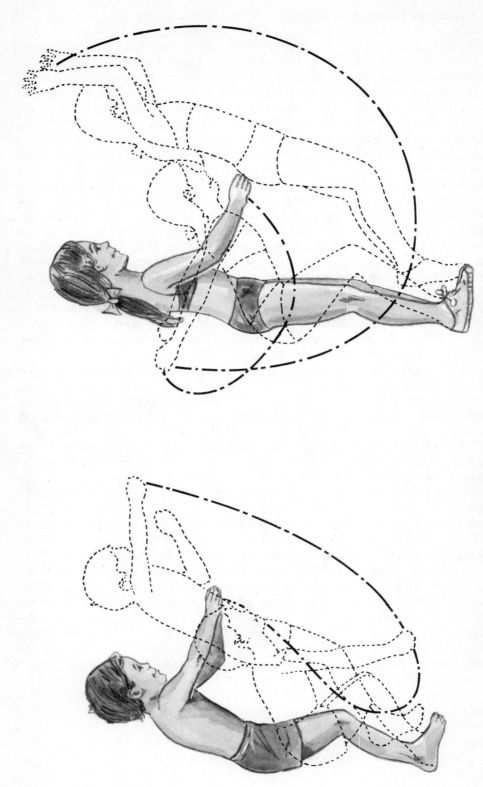

Figure 3-5 The differences in the preparatory arm action of the standing long jump. Which is more mature?

Zimmerman[22] studied college women who were classified as either skilled or unskilled broad jumpers. In the preparatory phase of the jump, skilled performers held the arms higher toward the rear of the body and then above the trunk as they began the movement. They held their arms high throughout the jump, whereas the nonskilled jumpers immediately lowered their arms and tended to swing them sideward as the legs came forward for landing. The skilled jumpers achieved full extension of their hips, knees, and ankles at takeoff, while the unskilled subjects were likely to hurry flexion of the hips and knees during the forward swing of the legs in the flight phase. Zimmerman further observed that good jumpers had a body inclination of approximately 45 degrees at takeoff.

Cooper and Glassow[7] discovered that the thigh position was a determining factor in the length of the reach at landing: "The more closely the thigh approaches the horizontal on landing, the longer is the reach." They further stated that "the horizontal position of the thighs changes the position of the center of gravity and permits that point to approach closer to the ground before the landing contact is made." In discussing the most efficient angle of takeoff, Cooper and Glassow noted that "whenever the takeoff is higher than the landing, as the center of gravity is in the standing broad jump, an angle of less than 45 degrees adds to the distance the projectile will travel."

During the early childhood period, the standing long jump progresses from an unstable movement that projects the body mainly in a vertical direction to a mature movement that efficiently uses the arms and legs in a coordinated horizontal jump. With development, the legs move simultaneously at takeoff and landing, and during the flight phase there is increased flexion at the hips and knees. As the child's balancing skills mature, the arms are used to increase momentum and stability in the preparatory crouch, takeoff, flight, and landing phases of the jump.

During the initial stage, the arms make only a limited contribution to the momentum of the jump. The degree of flexion of the legs during the preparatory crouch varies with each jump. The feet and legs do not work simultaneously during takeoff and landing. The extension of the lower extremities at takeoff is incomplete, as the jump is projected upward with little emphasis on the horizontal distance jumped. During the flight the legs are held stiff as the arms move to the side or the rear to maintain stability. At landing the legs are still stiff and therefore do not efficiently absorb the shock (Fig. 3–6).

The arms are utilized more productively during the elementary stage of the jumping pattern; they initiate the forward motion of the body at takeoff. The child also exhibits a more consistent preparatory crouch. There is a more complete extension of the lower extremities, and the angle of takeoff lowers, with greater emphasis on the horizontal component of the jump. The feet land simultaneously as the child falls rearward; and, like the infant, the child in the elementary stage tends to break the backward fall with the arms.

In the mature stage, the arms move high and toward the rear as the preparatory crouch is deepened to about a 90-degree angle. The arms initi-

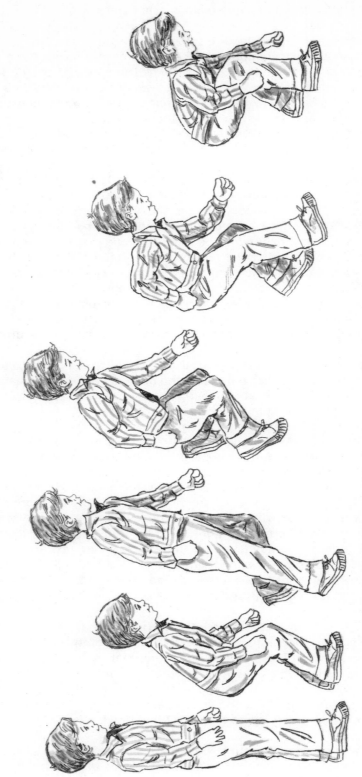

Figure 3–6 The initial stage of the jumping pattern. Note the movements of arms, feet, and legs.

ate the jumping action as they swing to a position high over the head and therefore add forward momentum to the jump. At the same time, there is a complete extension of the lower extremity that projects the body at approximately a 45-degree angle. The arms are held high throughout the flight, and the hips flex, bringing the thighs to a position parallel to the ground. At landing the body weight continues forward and downward as the arms reach forward.

SUMMARY

This chapter has reviewed the literature that deals with the acquisition of the fundamental locomotor patterns of walking, running, and jumping during early childhood. It may be concluded from this review that children refine these fundamental movements by passing through a series of increasingly complex stages.

The walking pattern is refined from a highly unstable act to an efficient movement. Running begins as a speeded-up, awkward walk and develops into a coordinated, rapid pattern. Jumping is characterized initially by an inability to maintain balance during flight and progresses to the point where longer and longer distances can be jumped. These changes in locomotor patterns are readily observable and may be utilized to evaluate a child's level of development.

BIBLIOGRAPHY

1. Anderson, Norma M., and Randall, Florence C.: An Experimental Study of Factors Which Influence Speed in Running. Unpublished master's thesis, University of Wisconsin, 1931, 52 pp.
2. Beck, Marjorie Catherine: The Path of the Center of Gravity During Running in Boys Grades One to Six. Unpublished doctoral dissertation, University of Wisconsin, 1965, 146 pp.
3. Broer, Marion: *Efficiency of Human Movement.* Philadelphia: W. B. Saunders Co., 1973, 453 pp.
4. Burnett, Carolyn N., and Johnson, Ernest W.: Development of gait in childhood: part 1 and part 2. *Developmental Medicine and Child Neurology, 13*:196–215, 1971.
5. Burnside, Lenoir H.: Coordination in the locomotion of infants. *Genetic Psychology Monographs, 2*:283–340, 1927.
6. Clouse, Florence C.: A Kinematic Analysis of the Development of the Running Pattern of Preschool Boys. Unpublished doctoral dissertation, University of Wisconsin, 1959, 260 pp.
7. Cooper, John M., and Glassow, Ruth B.: *Kinesiology.* St. Louis: C. V. Mosby Co., 1976, 352 pp.
8. Cratty, Bryant J.: *Perceptual and Motor Development in Infants and Children.* New York: Macmillan, 1970, 306 pp.
9. Dittmer, Joann A.: A Kinematic Analysis of the Development of Running Patterns of Grade School Girls and Certain Factors Which Distinguish Good and Poor Performance at Observed Ages. Unpublished master's thesis, University of Wisconsin, 1962, 196 pp.
10. Espenschade, Anna S., and Eckert, Helen M.: *Motor Development.* Columbus, Ohio: Charles E. Merrill, 1967, 280 pp.
11. Felton, Elvira A.: A Kinesiological Comparison of Good and Poor Performers in the Standing Broad Jump. Unpublished master's thesis, University of Wisconsin, 1960, 73 pp.

12. Fortney, Virginia L.: The Swinging Limb in Running of Boys Ages Seven Through Eleven. Unpublished master's thesis, University of Wisconsin, 1964, 166 pp.

13. Glassow, Ruth B., Halverson, Lolas, and Rarick, G. Lawrence: *Improvement of Motor Development and Physical Fitness in Elementary School Children,* Cooperative Research Project No. 696. Cooperative Research Program of the Office of Education, U.S. Department of Health, Education, and Welfare, and Wisconsin Alumni Research Foundation, 82 pp.

14. Godfrey, Barbara B., and Kephart, Newell C.: *Movement Patterns and Motor Education.* New York: Appleton-Century-Crofts, 1969, 310 pp.

15. Hillebrandt, F. A., Rarick, G. Lawrence, Glassow, Ruth B., and Carns, Marie L.: Physiological analysis of basic motor skills: I, growth and development of jumping. *American Journal of Physical Medicine, 40*:14–25, 1961.

16. McGraw, Myrtle B.: *The Neuromuscular Maturation of the Human Infant.* New York: Columbia University Press, 1943, 140 pp.

17. Rarick, G. Lawrence: *Motor Development During Infancy and Childhood.* Madison, Wis.: College Printing and Typing Co., 1961, 96 pp.

18. Shirley, Mary M.: *The First Two Years.* Minneapolis: University of Minnesota Press, 1931, 226 pp.

19. Sinclair, Caroline B.: *Movement of the Young Child: Ages Two to Six.* Columbus, Ohio: Charles E. Merrill, 1973, 128 pp.

20. Wellman, Beth L.: Motor achievement of preschool children. *Childhood Education, 13*:311–16, 1937.

21. Wickstrom, Ralph L.: *Fundamental Motor Patterns.* Philadelphia: Lea and Febiger, 1977, 209 pp.

22. Zimmerman, Helen M.: Characteristic Likenesses and Differences Between Skilled and Non-skilled Performance of the Standing Long Jump. Unpublished doctoral dissertation, University of Wisconsin, 1951, 155 pp.

CHAPTER 4

ACQUISITION OF FUNDAMENTAL MANIPULATIVE PATTERNS DURING EARLY CHILDHOOD

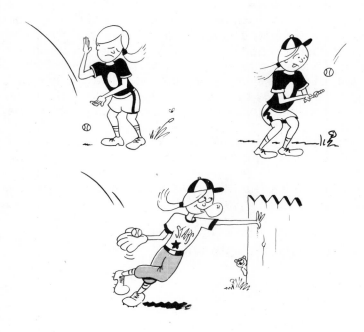

The Overhand Throwing Pattern
The Catching Pattern
The Kicking Pattern
Summary

During the early childhood period, fundamental manipulative patterns follow a path of development similar to that of the fundamental locomotor patterns. The ability to throw, catch, and kick objects progresses from early reflexive movements of the neonate to highly coordinated movement patterns of the elementary school—age child.

The early voluntary manipulative abilities of *reaching, grasping,* and *releasing* are important for the young child's exploration and understanding of the surrounding environment. The infant first tries to *reach* for an object with both arms in an uncoordinated and often unsuccessful corralling motion. The arms make a sweeping motion in an attempt to seize the object and draw it toward the body. With development of eye-hand coordination and improved muscular control, the infant gradually learns to use one arm in a well-directed reaching movement.

Early *grasping* movements are reflexive and involuntarily occur during the first few months of life when the infant's palm is stimulated. Initial voluntary attempts at grasping are palmar movements involving little control or use of the thumb. As the muscles of the fingers develop sufficiently, the thumb is gradually utilized in a more efficient pincer type of grasping action.

The ability to *release* an object is acquired after elementary forms of reaching and grasping have been learned. Halverson et al.[8] concluded that before 44 weeks of age, children cannot voluntarily release objects. Children pass through a period in which they can grasp an object but can release it only with the aid of a resisting surface. These rudimentary manipulative abilities are refined as muscle strength, coordination, and perception improve during infancy. By the time children enter early childhood, they have developed sufficient motor control to begin to explore and refine fundamental manipulative patterns.

This chapter reviews the literature on the acquisition of the manipulative patterns of throwing in an overhand manner, catching a small ball, and kicking a stationary ball. The ability to perform mature patterns is necessary for successful participation in complex sports such as baseball, softball, tennis, golf, and soccer.

THE OVERHAND THROWING PATTERN

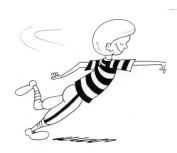

The overhand throw involves propelling an object into space by using the hands and arms in an over-the-shoulder pattern. Rarick[12] observed that because the throwing pattern requires the coordination of many body movements, children acquire the mature pattern slowly. By approximately 6

months of age, many children can throw from a sitting position, but only in an unrefined and awkward manner. It is not until a child is 1 year of age that he or she is able to control the direction of release.[7]

Guttridge[7] rated children's movement performance and noted that children between 2 and 3 years of age did not exhibit a good throwing pattern. However, 20 per cent of the 4-year-olds and 84 per cent of the 6-year-olds were rated as having proficient throwing ability.

Wild[16] conducted an in-depth study of the throwing pattern and its course of development in children. Thirty-two children served as subjects; they were grouped according to sex and age—a boy and a girl at each 6-month age level from 2 to 7 years of age and at each year level from 7 to 12 years of age. It was concluded that certain patterns for arm, body, and whole-throw components are typical of age. The results indicated that in developing the overhand throwing pattern, children pass through four progressive stages. Wild summarized these stages:

Stage I is characterized by typical anteroposterior movements. . . . The reverse movement of the arm is either sideways-upward or forward-upward usually too high above shoulder, elbow much flexed. With this reverse arm movement the trunk extends with dorsal flexion of ankles and carries the shoulders forward, and flexes forward with plantar flexion of ankles as the arm swings forward over the shoulder and down in front. Elbow extension starts early. Movements of body and arm are almost entirely in the anteroposterior plane over feet which remain in place; the body remains facing the direction of throw all the time; the arm is the initiating factor. There is trunk left rotation toward the end with the arm's forward reach.

Stage II, 3½ to 5 years, the whole body rotates right, then left above the feet; the feet remain together in place. The arm moves either in a high oblique plane above the shoulder or in a more horizontal plane, but with a forward downward follow-through. The elbow is much flexed; it may extend at once or later. The body changes its orientation and then reorientates to the throwing direction. The arm is the initiating factor.

Stage III, 5 to 6 years, marks the introduction of stepping; it is the right foot—step-forward throw. The weight is held back on the left rear foot as the spine rotates right and extends; the arm swings obliquely upward over the shoulder to a retracted position with elbow much flexed. The forward movements consist of a stepping forward with right foot, unilateral to the throwing arm, with spine left rotation, early turning of the whole body to a partial left facing and trunk forward flexion, while the arm swings forward either in an oblique-above-the-shoulder plane or in a sideways-around-the-shoulder plane, followed by a forward downward movement of follow-through. . . . This throw has both anteroposterior and horizontal features.

Stage IV is the left foot—step-forward throw with trunk rotation and horizontal adduction of the arm in the forward swing. This throw is the mature form and all boys from six and one-half years up have it. The girls have, in most cases, attained the body and foot movements, but incompletely developed forms of the arm movement.*

Wild[16] identified two distinct developmental trends. First, children's movement progresses from an anteroposterior plane to a horizontal plane; and second, with development, the base of support changes from a static to a shifting position.

Deach[5] indicated that in acquiring the mature throwing pattern, chil-

---

*From Wild, Monica: The behavior pattern of throwing and some observations concerning its course of development in children. *Research Quarterly, 116:22,* 1938. Used with permission.

dren between 2 and 6 years of age pass through four stages of development. Initially the elbow thrusts the ball forward in a high, short arch while the body faces the target and the feet are held close together. Trunk and leg movements are also limited, thus making the throw primarily an arm pattern. The second stage is characterized by restricted trunk and foot action on the throwing side. When there is a shift in body weight and the arms are moved in opposition to the trunk and feet, the third stage has been reached. In addition, the wrist completes the follow-through, and the fingers begin to control the direction of the ball. The final stage is typified by the placement of weight initially on the rear foot, the marked rotation of the trunk, and the dropping of the throwing shoulder. The arm moves in an overhand motion, and the weight is shifted to the forward foot. The shoulder of the throwing arm swings around to a position in line with the center of the target.

In summarizing the results of this portion of her study, Deach concluded that ". . . ability to execute a well-directed throw is accomplished through a continuous extension and sequent integration of motor coordinations involving first the arms then the trunk and finally the legs in a harmonious pattern."

After assessing the motor ability of young children, Keogh[11] concluded that many young children are unable to throw overhand in a consistent pattern. Many girls put the foot and arm on the same side forward when throwing. Keogh[11] also discussed fundamental motor tasks and indicated that throwing may be described in terms of movements of body parts. Initially the shoulder remains perpendicular to the target. With development, however, the shoulder rotates backward and then forward, thus marking the beginning of spinal rotation. The arm pattern changes similarly. Initially the elbow remains in front of the body for the throw, and the child pushes the ball; but as the arm pattern matures, the ball is brought behind the child's back before the throw. Whether the fingers at the point of release are spread or closed indicates a less mature or more mature pattern, respectively.

Cratty[4] identified five stages in the acquisition of a mature throwing pattern. At first the child attempts to push a ball along the floor. Next, using one hand and having little weight shift or shoulder rotation, the child throws the object. Later the head becomes stabilized as the object is thrown with greater shoulder rotation and a rudimentary forward shift in weight. This shift in weight gradually increases until the child steps forward on the foot that is on the same side as the throwing arm. The mature throwing action is characterized by a summation of forces that results in an efficient and coordinated pattern.

Brophy[1] studied the changes in body motion of eight college women who developed throwing skills. Motion pictures taken during three stages of learning the throw were analyzed. From these, she concluded that an improvement in throwing skills was accompanied by an increased range of movement in the arm and the trunk, a longer stride, and a better control of balance. She further determined that it was the amount of movement in the hip, rather than any other body segment, that correlated most closely with the degree of skill.

By analyzing the lever patterns of a boy and girl observed and filmed at 6-month intervals, Jones[10] was able to deduce that the most fundamental movement in the underarm and overarm throws was trunk rotation (Fig. 4–1A and B). She observed that throwing was most efficient when the motion of the hips, arms, and hands produced a series of four short levers contained within the longer lever of the arm.

During the early childhood period, children acquire a mature throwing form by passing through a series of complex stages. The progressive refinement of the throwing pattern may be summarized as follows. An inefficient arm action typifies the initial stage of the throwing pattern. Action is centered mainly at the elbow, which remains in front of the body throughout the throwing motion (Fig. 4–2A). The object is pushed forward as the fingers are spread at the point of release. There is limited rotation of the shoulder, and the child's body remains perpendicular to the target. As the arm follows through, there is a slight backward shift in weight. The feet remain stationary during the throwing motion.

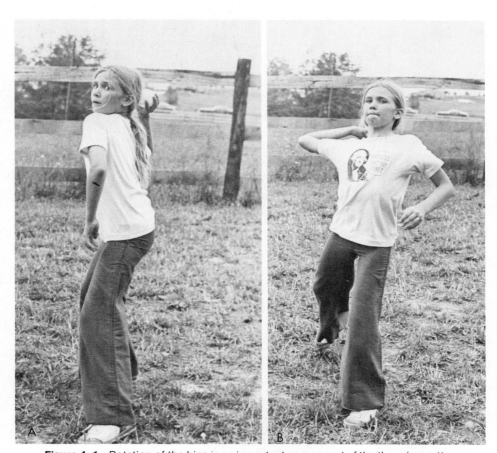

Figure 4–1 Rotation of the hips is an important component of the throwing pattern.

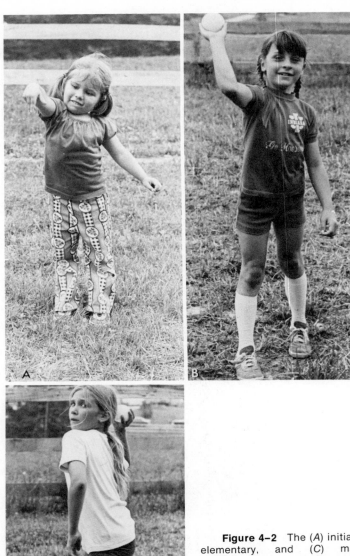

Figure 4–2 The (A) initial, (B) elementary, and (C) mature stages in the acquisition of the overhand throwing pattern. Attempt to identify the differences at each stage.

In the elementary stage of throwing, the arm, as it prepares to throw, swings increasingly from the shoulder to a position of flexion (Fig. 4–2B). The forward motion of the arm is high over the shoulder, and the follow-through is forward and down. The wrist completes the follow-through as the fingers gain increasing control over the release of the object. The trunk initially rotates to the throwing side during the preparatory swing of the arm and then flexes forward with the forward motion of the arm. At the same time, the weight is shifted to the front, and the child steps on the foot that is on the same side as the throwing arm.

A highly integrated throwing motion characterizes the mature stage of the throwing pattern. The arm is swung backward in preparation for the forward motion, and the trunk is rotated away from the target as the weight is shifted to the rear foot. The throwing shoulder drops slightly (Fig. 4–2C). As the arm begins its forward motion, the trunk rotates away from the throwing side through the hips, spine, and shoulders; and as the weight is shifted forward with a step on the nonthrowing side, momentum is added to the throw. During the throw, the elbow moves forward and leads the hand, causing a whipping action of the upper arm. The arm adducts horizontally as the object is released from the fingers. At the release, the shoulders swing to a position perpendicular to the target, and the arm follows through downward across the body to the opposite knee in a thumb-down position.

THE CATCHING PATTERN

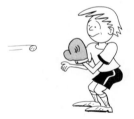

Catching is a fundamental movement pattern in which the momentum of a thrown object is brought under control by the arms and the hands. The acquisition of catching skills follows the same basic development as other fundamental movement patterns during early childhood.

Wellman[14] studied the motor achievements of preschool children and identified three levels of development in the catching pattern. At the first level, children younger than 3½ years of age who are trying to catch a ball hold their arms straight and stiff at the elbows and in front of the body. At the second level (around age 4) the child's hands open to receive the object, although the arms remain in a stiff position. The final level is characterized by a change in arm position. The arms are now held bent and to the sides of the body, and they "give" in order to absorb the impact of the object.

In describing the development of the catching pattern, Espenschade and Eckert[6] identified similar stages of development. In the early stage the arms are held outstretched and stiff, and there is little effort to adjust body position to the flight of the ball. The arms, used to make a basket type of catch, usually fail to catch the ball. With time and practice, the arms become more relaxed, and the child catches the ball by scooping it up against his body. Later the hands are held together at the wrist and used in a vise-like grip. The elbows are held at either side of the body so that they may give as the arms absorb the object's momentum. In the mature pattern the hands are cupped together with either the thumbs or the little fingers in opposition, depending upon the position of the tossed ball.

In a study of the relationship between chronological age and motor skill development, Guttridge[7] determined that catching proficiency increased with age. Twenty-nine per cent of the 4-year-old children studied were proficient catchers; 56 per cent of the 5-year-olds were rated as good; and 63 per cent of the 6-year-olds had a well-developed catching pattern. She found that there are definite stages in the development of a good catching form, depending on the methods used to catch a ball. In early attempts, the whole body tries to clasp the ball. As development progresses, the arms are used less in the movement, and gradually the ball is caught between the palms of the hands. Guttridge also reported that the size of the ball played an important role in a child's catching ability. Some 6-year-old children were able to catch a 12-inch ball, whereas 50 per cent achieved success with an 8-inch ball and 55 per cent were successful with a 6-inch ball. Eighty-two per cent of the children observed could catch a 5-inch ball.

Cratty[3] noted that catching behavior passes through several stages. During the earliest stage the child passively waits for the ball to be placed in his arms, which are held in a cradle position. In the second stage the child holds the arms stiff and in front of the body. Finally the child holds his arms relaxed and at his sides before he attempts to catch the ball.

In analyzing motion pictures, Deach[5] observed that there seem to be two distinct patterns of catching. She noted that children at first used their arms and bodies to catch the ball. With maturity, however, they controlled the ball with their fingers.

Deach summarized five stages of development in catching a small ball thrown at chest level. Children first exhibit a defensiveness that is characterized by tenseness of the body or protection of the head with the arms and hands. There is no effort made to step forward or to catch the ball. Children in the second stage try to catch the ball but are unsuccessful. The catching action of the arms consists of a scooping motion. As the catch is attempted, there is a definite step forward but the timing is poor; thus the ball either falls away or hits the body and bounces away. The arms are held tense, and there is still a slight defensiveness present during this stage. In the next phase of development, the arms are extended forward and held fairly close together. As the ball drops in front of the body, the arms are clasped to the chest. The fingers are spread and extended and are slow to function in completing the catch. The fourth stage functions as a transition between the clumsy arm and body catch and the efficient finger catch. The timing of the arms and fingers is inaccurate, and the child is unable to adjust his body position to varied ball positions. The final stage is characterized by successful catches with the fingers and hands. The body is brought into a position of readiness; the hands and arms may be extended forward, or they may move from the sides. The catch is timed to meet the ball, and the arms give to absorb the force of the ball. The fingers initially make the catch and the hands then assist.

Victors[13] evaluated the catching behavior of 7- and 9-year-old boys, with each group consisting of five good and five poor performers. She observed that the 9-year-olds most often completed hand closure with both hands simultaneously. The younger group tended to exhibit an uneven grasp, with one hand generally closing more rapidly.

Wickstrom[15] discovered that if a ball is thrown to a child too early in his development, there may be no effective catching response. At 2 years of age, the child will let the ball strike him in the chest before he attempts to catch it. A 3-year-old child usually needs to be told how to position his arms before receiving the ball.

It may be concluded that there are several distinct stages in the acquisition of the mature catching pattern and that a child exhibits an initial, an elementary, and a mature catching pattern during the period of early childhood.

In the initial stage of the catching pattern, the child displays an avoidance reaction by turning the face away or by utilizing the arms for protection as the ball is thrown. Held with elbows extended toward the thrower, the arms do not move to "scoop" the ball until contact is made. The palms of the hands are up, and the fingers are extended and tense (Fig. 4–3A). There is very little use of the hands as the child attempts to trap the ball to his chest. The catching action is usually poorly timed and inefficient.

In the elementary stage, the avoidance reaction has been eliminated, and the child's eyes begin to follow the path of the ball. The lower arms are held to the front of the body with an approximate 90-degree bend at the elbows, which the child keeps close to his sides. The palms of the hands are held directly opposite to each other and perpendicular to the ground (Fig. 4–3B). The fingers are extended as the hands attempt to grasp the ball in a poorly timed motion; the hands often miss the ball, and the arms then must secure the ball to the body. By the time the child has acquired a mature catching pattern, his eyes follow the ball from the time of its release to when it is caught. The arms are bent and held relaxed at the child's sides or held with the upper arms directly in front of the body to await the ball. The arms adjust to the flight of the ball and give to help absorb the ball's momentum. The hands are held in a cupped position with the thumbs (when the ball is tossed above the waist) or little fingers (when the ball is tossed below the waist) in opposition (Fig. 4–3C). The hands and fingers close around the ball in a coordinated and well-timed motion.

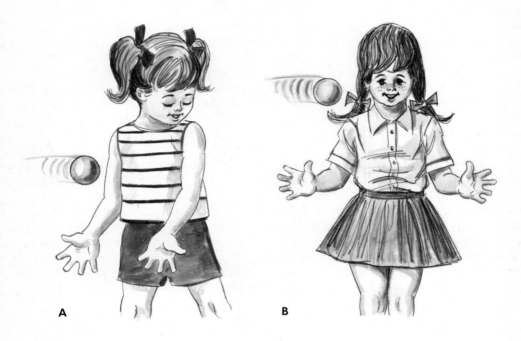

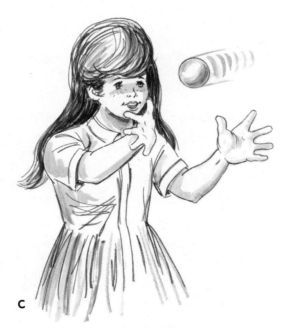

Figure 4–3 Various hand positions of the catching pattern in the (A) initial, (B) elementary, and (C) mature stages.

THE KICKING PATTERN

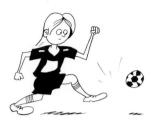

Kicking is a manipulative pattern in which the action of the legs and feet imparts force to an object. To date, research on the progressive development of kicking is limited. However, Deach[5] studied the kicking behavior of children between 2 and 6 years of age and concluded that "the elements in the form of a highly skilled kick seem to appear in such a sequence that there are different stages of progress toward the ability to execute a well-coordinated kick."

Deach analyzed the kicking of a stationary ball from a starting position immediately behind it and discovered that there were four stages in the acquisition of the kicking pattern. The first stage was characterized by little activity of the trunk and arms, and legs. The free foot was placed behind the ball, and the leg swung forward from the hip. The body remained erect with the arms held at the sides. There was no backswing before the ball was kicked and only a short forward swing in the follow-through to the left (Fig. 4–4).

In the second stage, the child began to utilize the arms. The arm on the preferred side tended to swing forward and backward while the opposite arm moved from a backward or sideward position to a forward position once the kick was completed. The knee was bent, and the kick was made from the knee with the follow-through fairly high as the body bent at the waist.

During the third stage, the backward movement of the leg in the preparatory phase of the kick was initiated at the hip. The body did not shift forward enough to allow full extension of the hip, and as a result, the knee bent to increase the backward movement of the lower leg. The child's weight was placed on the ball of the support foot, and the support leg bent as the kicking leg started its forward movement. Upon contact with the ball, the kicking leg extended and then continued its forward swing in a complete follow-through.

A child who developed his kicking pattern to the final stage utilized a full leg swing from the hips along with an increased arm movement. The trunk flexed at the waist, and the support foot rose on its toes during the follow-through. Contact was usually made slightly under the ball so that it was lifted in flight.

In reviewing the work of Deach, Wickstrom[15] noted that the children who were studied tended to retract the kicking leg after completion of the

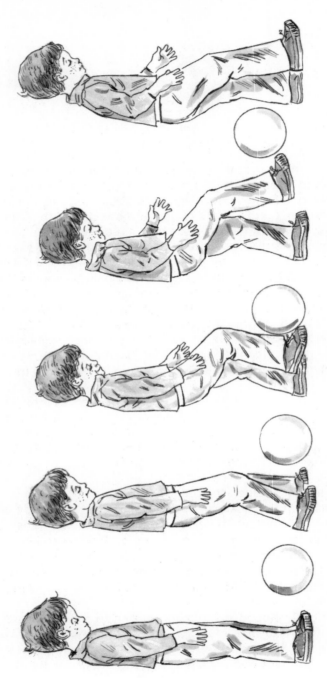

Figure 4–4 Initial stage in the development of the kicking pattern. Note the limited use of the arms and legs.

kick: "This tendency to withdraw the kicking leg is a clearly identifiable aspect of the developmental form of kicking." He referred to a child's early attempts as "kicking at" the ball rather than the more mature form of "kicking through" it.

Halverson and Robertson[9] showed that as the backswing increases, the follow-through must also increase in order to absorb the force of the kicking leg. As the force of the kick becomes greater, the arms are used more to maintain balance.

Although research on the development of the kicking pattern is limited, the acquisition of the mature kicking pattern may be summarized as follows.

Initial attempts at kicking a stationary ball are characterized by relatively little action of the arms and the trunk. The trunk remains erect as the arms are held to the child's sides. There is no backward movement of the kicking leg in preparation for the forward swing, and the follow-through is limited. The swing of the leg is poorly timed, and the child may skim the top of the ball with his foot or miss the ball altogether.

During the elementary stage, the arms are held outward for stability and the leg action is centered mainly at the knee. The leg flexes to the rear at the knee and quickly extends forward to hit the ball. After contact with the ball, the leg continues its forward swing in a short and limited follow-through.

A child's arms swing in opposition to the legs during the mature stage of the kicking pattern. With only a slight knee flexion, the kicking leg swings mainly from the hip and moves through a large arc. The support leg bends slightly at contact. During the high follow-through, the support foot rises to its toes as the child bends slightly forward at the waist.

SUMMARY

This chapter has reviewed the literature on the sequential acquisition during early childhood of the fundamental manipulative patterns of throwing, striking, catching, and kicking. With the refinement of physical abilities, children develop more efficient, mature manipulative patterns.

Manipulative patterns appear to develop in a sequence similar to fundamental locomotor patterns. Throwing and striking are refined from a simple arm action to a well-timed coordination of many body segments. In acquiring a mature catching form, children learn to use their hands and fingers. The leg swings from the knee during the early stages of the kicking pattern, but with maturity and practice, the swinging action is centered at the hip for increased leverage. Like the changes in locomotor patterns reviewed in the previous chapter, the changes that take place in the development of the manipulative patterns may also be used to assess a child's developmental level.

BIBLIOGRAPHY

1. Brophy, Kathleen J.: A Kinesiological Study of the Improvement in Motor Skill. Unpublished doctoral dissertation, University of Wisconsin, 1948, 170 pp.

2. Corbin, Charles: *A Textbook of Motor Development.* Dubuque, Iowa: William C. Brown, 1973, 184 pp.
3. Cratty, Bryant J.: *Perceptual and Motor Development in Infants and Children.* New York: Macmillan, 1970, 315 pp.
4. Cratty, Bryant J.: *Remedial Motor Activity for Children:* Philadelphia: Lea and Febiger, 1975, 327 pp.
5. Deach, Dorothy F.: Genetic Development of Motor Skills in Children Two Through Six Years of Age. Unpublished doctoral dissertation, University of Michigan, 1951, 401 pp.
6. Espenschade, Anna S., and Eckert, Helen M.: *Motor Development.* Columbus, Ohio: Charles E. Merrill, 1967, 280 pp.
7. Guttridge, Mary V.: A study of motor achievements of young children. *Archives of Psychology, 244*:1–178, 1939.
8. Halverson, H. M., et al.: An experimental study of prehension in infants by means of systematic cinema records. *Genetic Psychology Monographs, 10*:107, 1931.
9. Halverson, Lolas E., and Robertson, M. A.: A Study of Motor Pattern Development in Young Children. Presented at the National Convention of the American Association for Health, Physical Education, and Recreation, Chicago, March 18–22, 1966.
10. Jones, Fredda Goodwin: A Descriptive and Mechanical Analysis of Throwing Skills of Children. Unpublished master's thesis, University of Wisconsin, 1951, 94 pp.
11. Keogh, Jack: Motor Performance of Elementary School Children. Los Angeles: University of California Department of Physical education, 1965.
12. Rarick, G. Lawrence: *Motor Development During Infancy and Childhood.* Madison, Wis.: College Printing and Typing Co., 1961, 96 pp.
13. Victors, Evelyn E.: A Cinematographical Analysis of Catching Behavior of a Selected Group of Seven and Nine Year Old Boys. Unpublished doctoral dissertation, University of Wisconsin, 1961, 139 pp.
14. Wellman, Beth L.: Motor achievement of pre-school children. *Childhood Education, 13*:311–16, 1937.
15. Wickstrom, Ralph L.: *Fundamental Motor Patterns.* Philadelphia: Lea & Febiger, 1977, 209 pp.
16. Wild, Monica: The behavior pattern of throwing and some observations concerning its course of development in children. *Research Quarterly, 9*:20–24, 1938.

PROGRAM DESIGN

SECTION CONCEPTS

1. The motor development program should be planned in four steps that include (1) pre-program planning, (2) pre-program assessment, (3) determination of curriculum content, and (4) post-program assessment.
2. Systematic observation can be utilized to evaluate efficiently a child's ability to perform mature fundamental movement patterns.
3. The manner in which the program is organized and implemented will, to a large degree, determine the success of the program.
4. Fundamental movements can be taught to children by using either direct or indirect teaching styles, depending upon the needs of the children being served.

CHAPTER 5

A MODEL FOR ENHANCING FUNDAMENTAL MOVEMENT PATTERNS

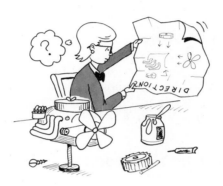

Once the decision has been made to provide children with activities to improve their fundamental movement abilities, the teacher becomes involved in a number of important procedures for program development. Each of the following four steps is necessary for insuring the operation of a worthwhile program that is geared to the developmental needs and interests of the children for whom the program is intended. Careful planning that includes determination of the aims and objectives of the movement pattern program is the first step in the process. Second, the children's level of psychomotor, cognitive, and affective functioning must be carefully evaluated. The third step involves outlining the program content, namely the specific objectives and the appropriate movement experiences necessary to satisfy these objectives. The fourth and final step is post-program assessment; it is crucial that the children in the movement pattern program be periodically evaluated in order to judge whether the specific objectives and movement experiences are fulfilling their needs.

Each of these four steps will be detailed in this chapter. Particular attention will be given to the importance of pre-program planning, pre-program assesment, curriculum content, and post-program assessment in establishing and maintaining an effective motor development program.

PRE-PROGRAM PLANNING

Before embarking on the development of any curriculum, whether it be in motor development, science, or mathematics, it is important to determine just what the program is all about. This is generally done through a concise statement of program aims and general objectives.

DETERMINE THE AIMS OF THE PROGRAM

The aims of the motor development program are the long-term goals expressed in very general terms. The aims of any motor development program should center on helping children learn to move and helping them learn through movement.

Learning to Move. The primary aim of the movement program at all levels is helping children and adults learn how to use their bodies more efficiently and effectively. Parents are concerned with helping their infant develop a wide variety of rudimentary movement abilities through a combination of maturation and environmental opportunity. The toddler learns to move by acquiring a variety of movement patterns at the initial level. The preschooler upgrades these same movement patterns into more efficient forms, and the primary grade child further refines them. The intermediate and upper elementary grade child learns to move in different and often more complex ways than his or her younger counterpart; at this age, the child begins to apply fundamental movements to various sport and dance skills. As the child moves with greater efficiency and control in sport-related skills, he begins to learn more about his physical abilities (Fig. 5–1). The junior and senior high school student continues to learn to move with higher degrees of form, skill, and accuracy, and generally at this age begins to narrow the scope of active involvement in physical activities to two or three favorites. The adult also keeps learning to move while engaging in physical activities on either a recreational or a competitive basis.

For the fully functioning individual, learning to move is a lifelong process of movement skill acquisition, adaptation, and change. Helping the

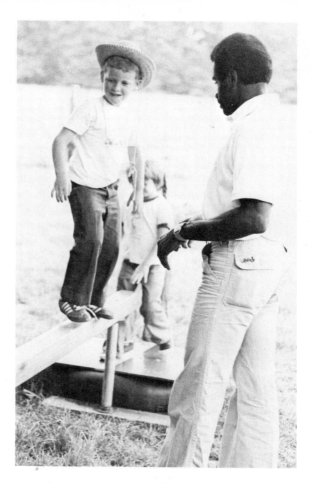

Figure 5–1 Developing stability skills in learning to move.

individual to move is the primary aim of any quality program of motor development at any level as well as the primary reason for the quality physical educator's existence in our nation's public schools. Learning to move is an important part of a person's total education because it helps the individual become and remain active, energetic, and functioning to the extent of his capacity.

Learning Through Movement. When we speak of learning through movement, which is secondary to learning to move, we are generally talking about the potential for using movement as a developer and reinforcer of various cognitive and affective concepts. Infants and toddlers use movement as their primary method of information gathering. The environment is experienced both through the senses and through active exploration. Movement is at the core of early perceptual and motor development of toddlers and preschoolers. Primary and intermediate grade children use movement in more subtle ways as an information-gathering device. Through the medium of movement they learn about their bodies and experience interpersonal relationships. For junior and senior high school–age youngsters, active involvement in sport and dance activities helps them gain information about themselves in terms of personal strengths and weaknesses, emotional stability, peer interaction, strategy implementation, knowledge of rules, and so forth. Because interaction with the environment through recreational activities continues throughout life, active adults also keep learning through movement.

Learning *through* movement arises from learning to move (Fig. 5–2). The quality motor development program that stresses the development of one's psychomotor abilities also makes positive contributions to the individual's cognitive and affective development. How strongly learning through movement is emphasized, however, depends on the program objectives, through which the aims of the motor development program are achieved.

DETERMINE THE GENERAL OBJECTIVES

The next step in planning a program of physical activities to enhance fundamental movement is determining the general objectives of the program.

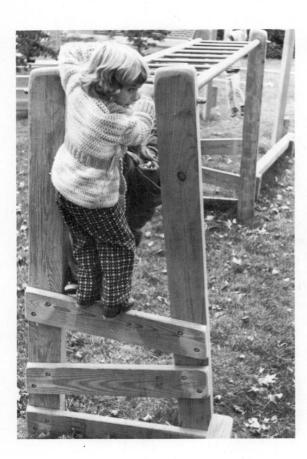

Figure 5–2 Knowing our limitations by learning through movement. (Courtesy of Creative Playgrounds Corp., Terre Haute, Ind. Used with permission.)

The motor development program may emphasize one or both of the following general objectives, depending upon the psychomotor needs of the children to be served.

1. Developmental Objective. To provide children at the preschool and primary grade levels with a program of movement experiences designed to give them sufficient opportunity to develop mature and efficient movement patterns.

2. Remedial Objective. To provide children at the middle and upper elementary grade levels with the opportunity to participate in a motor development program designed to correct any lag in the attainment of mature movement patterns.

The developmental program objective stated previously can usually be accomplished by giving young children a properly planned physical education program that includes experiences in fundamental movement. These movement experiences should teach children how their bodies move as well as the potentials and limitations of their bodies. This program should stress the development of fundamental movement, perceptual motor skills, and rhythmical abilities. The use of games and sports at this level should be limited and utilized only on a selected basis.

The remedial program is designed for children who have passed beyond the critical period of early childhood without having developed mature movement abilities. These children should be identified early and then grouped according to their motor needs. This type of program should focus primarily on developing locomotor and manipulative patterns as well as on improving the components of fundamental movement, such as stability, flexibility, strength, and coordination. The appropriate prescriptive movement experiences should be developed and then presented to children in a more concentrated manner than the developmental program. Therefore, the individual may wish to provide several lessons designed to enhance one specific movement pattern, such as running.

The motor development program at the elementary level may be remedial or developmental or a combination of the two. The objective of the program depends upon the needs of the students, the concerns and competencies of the teachers, and the facilities and materials available to the program.

Although it is easy to justify the need for physical education at the preschool and elementary levels, many children are not provided with this type of program. Thus concerned individuals working with elementary-age children may be called upon to plan motor development programs. In doing so, these individuals should familiarize themselves with the process of skill acquisition as well as with activities designed to enhance development of motor skills.

A motor development program may be initiated with little regard for facilities and equipment. All too often we hear the excuse, "We can't do that; we have no gymnasium equipment." Various movement experiences can be designed to fit safely within the limitations of the program. Most activities can be adapted for performance in a restricted space. For example, children can attempt to kick balloons instead of playground balls. The movement pattern

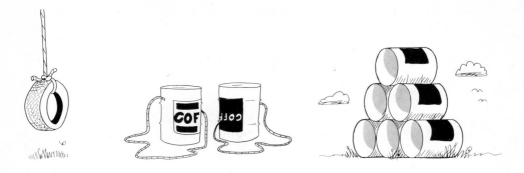

is similar, but the activity is structured so that participants are not endangered.

Numerous companies are in the business of supplying schools with equipment for motor development or physical education classes. Most of this equipment is highly priced, and even schools with large budgets have difficulty supplying enough commercially produced equipment for each student. However, there are several excellent texts available (they may be found in the bibliography of this chapter) that give directions for making equipment out of items normally thrown away. Students can even help to make equipment for their own program, and a large amount of material can be accumulated at little cost. Appendix B contains a list of easily made, inexpensive equipment that is ideal for providing children with appropriate movement experiences.

PRE-PROGRAM ASSESSMENT

Upon observation of the movement patterns of boys and girls, it soon becomes apparent that not all children, even those of the same age, are at the same level of development. As has been discussed previously, environmental opportunities, timely experiences, and motivation play a key role in the development and refinement of fundamental movement patterns. Because of the unique hereditary background of each child and its intricate interaction with environment, experience, and motivation, we typically see a variety of differences *between children, within children,* and *within patterns.*

Differences between children can readily be observed in the typical elementary classroom, where we see some children functioning at the initial level, some at the elementary level, and still others at the mature level in the development of their movement pattern. More from expediency than from ignorance of child development, children are often grouped and instructed in physical education as if they were all at the same level of motor development. This would indeed be a pleasant situation if it were so. Imagine having a class of 30 children all at the same level of motor development; there would be no need to individualize instruction or account for differences between children. The chances of this occurring, however, is no less remote than the chance of having a class of 30 students all at the same level of cognitive or affective development. We must recognize that the unique background of each child is important to the progress he makes in learning and mastering movement abilities. Methods of instruction and the content of lessons must reflect an understanding of and appreciation for differences between children.

There are also *differences within children* that the astute teacher will recognize. Some children may display mature locomotor behavior in running and jumping but may be at only the initial or elementary level in the manipulative activities of throwing and catching. The comment "he throws like a girl," although unfortunate, is all too often true. Many girls and women, because of lack of opportunity for experience, display immature throwing and catching patterns. However, they often show maturity in running, jumping, and skipping because of encouragement in these areas during childhood. Opportunity for practice, instruction, and motivation help determine the degree to which an individual develops and refines the numerous locomotor and manipulative patterns of movement. The competitive athlete who is required to specialize at an early age often manifests splinter skills. In other words, he may be mature in the skills characteristic of the particular sport but less than mature in a variety of others.

The careful observer of children can also note that there are often *differences within patterns.* For example, in throwing, the arms may perform at the mature level, the trunk at the initial level, and the legs at the elementary level. Although differences within patterns are not as common or readily observable as differences between children and within children, they do exist. The job of the instructor is to help the child develop the less mature components of the pattern.

It is important that we recognize the existence of differences between children, within children, and within patterns. All too often we have failed to do so and have glossed over the acquisition of fundamental movement patterns in a few short lessons or in a few pages in the voluminous literature on child development. If children are to develop their movement abilities in an orderly, sequential, and sound manner, we must recognize the individuality of the learner and the importance of acquiring mature patterns of movement that serve as the basis for achieving sport skills.

Movement activities that help a child progress from one level of motor development to the next must be viewed both from a psychomotor perspective and from a cognitive and affective perspective. This is a crucial point that must be constantly taken into consideration when dealing with children; it is both unwise and unfair to require them to take part in activities that are consistently above or beneath their developmental level. Apathy, frustration, boredom, and a lack of self-confidence may result from such a requirement. For example, Mark, a 9-year-old of normal intelligence who is entering the fourth grade, is described by both his teachers and peers as "awkward," "clumsy," or a "real klutz." He functions at no better than an elementary level in several movement patterns. In order to help Mark attain greater efficiency in his movement behavior, we need to involve him in a series of activities that are appropriate for his level of psychomotor development. However, it would be imprudent to encourage activities that, although developmentally sound for Mark, are not suited to his cognitive and affective level, given his age and normal intelligence. Loosely structured exploratory activities involving such things as animal walks, story dramatization, and games with low organization like "Duck-Duck Goose," or "Brownies and Fairies" would be disastrous for Mark. He would soon reject them as being for "babies" and become bored and totally disinterested in the program.

It would be much better to devise a series of movement experiences for Mark or any similar youngster, including the gifted child who is neither at nor near the expected level of development, that accounts for all aspects of his development. In doing so it becomes possible to end the cycle of frustration, failure, and rejection of physical activity that follows from inappropriate experiences. Only when the movement experiences are appropriate can we be sure that the needs and interests of children are truly being satisfied. We can serve children by structuring activities in such a way that excitement, interest, and challenge are retained while more mature patterns are being established. For example, in the game of Tee Ball, a modified version of baseball in which the ball is struck from a batting tee rather than hit after being hurled by a pitcher, the child still has an opportunity to take part in a type of baseball game but also has a greater chance of being successful in hitting the ball. At the same time, the child gains valuable experience in developing a more mature striking pattern.

STAGES IN PSYCHOMOTOR DEVELOPMENT

In Chapters 3 and 4, literature on the development of a variety of locomotor and manipulative patterns was reviewed and summarized. From this review we were able to see that there is a developmental progression for each of the patterns discussed; this progression was divided into three stages of development—the *initial, elementary,* and *mature.* Studies on the acquisition of fundamental movement patterns support their developmental nature. That is, these patterns do not suddenly appear in their mature form but rather are learned and refined through the complex interaction of maturation and experience. Maturation alone does not account for the acquisition of mature patterns; experience plays a vital role, particularly during the crucial early childhood years.

Motor development progresses quickly as the child begins to explore the movement capabilities of his body. Rarick states that once the child enters the period of early childhood, "development of basic motor abilities is so rapid that most of the fundamental movement patterns are quite well established before the child enters school."[9] If the child fails to keep pace with others in his development, he is then unable to participate on the same level as his peers because of deficiencies in the performance of various patterns. Espenschade and Eckert stated that "such an effect may snowball in that the child's inability to play on equal terms with others further limits opportunities for practice and so he falls still further behind."[4] It is, therefore, important that children be offered carefully planned motor development programs that give them experiences to help improve their movement patterns.

During early childhood, children pass through stages of development at various rates. A significant number are late in forming refined, efficient patterns of movement. They may pass through the stages more slowly than may normally be expected, or their progress may be arrested at a level lower than that characteristic of their age and maturity. It is, therefore, important that children's level of motor functioning be assessed early. If development is delayed beyond the critical period of early childhood, the child may never achieve mature patterns without loss of time and considerable difficulty in terms of effort and individual instruction.

The degree to which a child or group of children has developed fundamental movement abilities may be assessed by using the instrument discussed in detail in Chapter 6. This observational technique, designed to help the observer evaluate the development of fundamental movement patterns, provides a quick and easy way of collecting subjective data about a particular child or group of children. The reader is referred to Chapter 6 for an in-depth discussion of this tool and how it is used.

There are a number of other checklists and movement pattern inventories available.[6, 10] Although they have made valuable contributions to the study of motor development, they tend to be cumbersome to use and difficult to interpret. The observational technique in this text attempts to avoid these pitfalls. It enables the observer to determine the child's unique profile of ability in a variety of carefully researched locomotor and manipulative patterns. The profile provides the user with a general idea of the level at which the child is functioning, whether it be the initial, elementary, or mature stage, or a combination of the three. The information gained from this assessment inventory should be considered in conjunction with information about the cognitive and affective maturity of the learner.

LEVELS OF COGNITIVE AND AFFECTIVE DEVELOPMENT

When selecting movement experiences we must be concerned with their cognitive and affective appropriateness as well as their psychomotor suitability. The age-appropriateness of a particular activity or type of movement activity is determined by the usual level of cognitive and affective maturity of children at any given age. It must be remembered that there is often considerable variability in maturity *between* children. It is wrong to assume that all children in the period of early childhood have reached the same level of cognitive and affective development. Yet we often assume this when programming movement experiences for them. We tend to group young children according to age only and program experiences for them as if they were identical to one another, but this is done in violation of all that is known about children and how they develop during this period.

Literature about the growth and development of children is abundant and clearly validates the concept of progressive levels of cognitive and affective behaviors as well as of psychomotor development. The works of Piaget,[8] Erikson,[3] and Gesell,[5] probably the best known on the subject, are among many that support the idea of a sequential acquisition of more mature forms of functioning. The complex interaction of heredity with environment accounts for a rather rigid *sequence* of acquisition of these forms as well as for variability in the *rate* of development between children.

Perhaps it would be wise to classify movement activities on the basis of the *typical* maturity level of the children for whom they are intended. The following is a list of guidelines for structuring movement experiences for both the developmental and remedial programs.

Experiences in the *developmental program* are geared to the cognitive and affective level of the typical child 3 through 6 years of age. Movement experiences designed to enhance fundamental movement should:

1. Provide plenty of opportunity for structured and unstructured motor play involving the whole body.
2. Use a variety of movement exploration and guided discovery techniques that permit and encourage children to perform various movement patterns.
3. Utilize individual activities and gradually introduce the children to group activities and encourage group interaction.
4. Emphasize creative expression and exploration in an atmosphere of love, acceptance, and success.
5. Encourage children to *think* before, during, and after the performance of a fundamental movement.
6. Include numerous experiences for developing component skills of fundamental movement, such as stability and flexibility, as well as perceptual-motor activities.
7. Make use of the child's vivid imagination through drama, mimetics, and story plays.
8. Encourage children to "show and tell" others what they can do to help overcome shyness.
9. Use a multisensory approach in the presentation of movement experiences.
10. Allow for individual differences between children and stress individual and, to a degree, group progress.

Experiences in the *remedial program* are geared to the cognitive and affective level of the typical child 7 through 10 years of age. Remedial movement experiences designed to enhance fundamental movement at this level should:

1. Stress application of patterns of movement to a wide variety of sport-related skills.
2. Introduce children to a wide range of activities that lead up to a variety of individual, dual, and team sports requiring fundamental movement.

3. Emphasize form, skill, and accuracy in the performance of fundamental movement patterns.
4. Utilize problem-solving techniques at the initial stages of learning, but generally rely more on direct methods of teaching.
5. Permit children to combine several movement patterns into a more complex motor skill.
6. Encourage children to select the best ways of performing specific movements in an atmosphere of helpfulness and encouragement.
7. Instruct children to practice the correct movement form on their own outside class time.
8. Introduce basic team strategies along with concepts of teamwork, fair play, and ethical behavior.
9. Do not separate boys and girls for instruction periods, but recognize their needs to learn with each other and to accept one another.
10. Keep competition at the children's level, and provide opportunities for intramural activities for all children.

From a careful reading of each of the program suggestions presented for both the developmental and remedial programs, a few general principles should emerge. Namely, that *as we progress from one program to the other,* there is:

1. A move from the simple to the relatively complex in the teaching of movement patterns and skills.
2. A move from general to more specific types of activities.
3. A gradually increased emphasis on form, accuracy, and improved performance levels.
4. A transition from open-ended movement exploration and guided discovery teaching techniques to more teacher-directed combination and selection experiences.
5. A transition from the development of mature movement patterns to the development of basic sport skills.
6. Increased affective maturity resulting in a transition from individual and small group activities to team-oriented activities.
7. Increased cognitive maturity permitting greater exploration of the reasons behind the performance of movement patterns and skills. Therefore, mechanics, performance potentials, rules, and strategy are gradually more emphasized.

Only when we recognize children's cognitive and affective development as well as their psychomotor development can we select and implement movement experiences that are sound. Then we are faced with the critical question of just *how* we can do this.

Children's cognitive and affective level of development may be formally assessed. There are a multitude of tests that measure intelligence, academic achievement, personality traits, and self concept.[2] It would, however, be unreasonable to assume that the teacher has the results of formal test scores available on an individual basis. The motor development specialist must generally rely on characteristic behaviors of children at a given age level. A broad understanding of *typical* behavior patterns of children at various age levels and careful observation of the specific children in one's charge make it possible for the teacher to structure appropriate movement experiences for individuals or groups.

Suitable experiences based on the developmental level of children should be selected and incorporated into the motor development program. For example, 5-year-olds are typically at the elementary stage in the acquisition of their fundamental movement patterns. Knowing this, we should be able to prescribe appropriate experiences. Some children, however, may be at the mature stage in their pattern development, so we need to be sure that the activities we structure for them continually refine these patterns and promote greater skill development. Some 5- to 7-year-olds may still be at the initial stage of their pattern development in one or more movements. We need to recognize this and provide them with the types of experiences that will help them upgrade their skill without sacrificing challenge, excitement, and fun.

CURRICULUM CONTENT

Once we have assessed the level of psychomotor development as well as determined the children's cognitive and affective level, we can design learning experiences to meet their needs. Curriculum planning involves determining the specific objectives as well as the individual learning experiences of the program.

DETERMINE SPECIFIC OBJECTIVES

A great deal has been said and written about specific objectives over the past several years. Behavioral objectives, one form of specific objective, have come into vogue in recent years, and the reader is referred to excellent

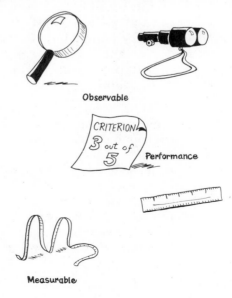

Observable

CRITERION 3 out of 5 / Performance

Measurable

texts by Bloom[1] and Mager[7] on the subject. Briefly, behavioral objectives are performance objectives. They are (1) observable, (2) measurable, and (3) establish the criterion for performance. Behavioral objectives help us to keep the goals of our lesson continually in focus. It is not necessary to state a specific objective for each activity in which a child may participate. One behavioral objective may suffice for a series of movement experiences geared to achieving a specific end. For example, a typical objective is to be able to run a distance of 25 yards utilizing a mature pattern that involves proper use of the arms, trunk, and legs throughout. Each specific objective should be selected on the basis of the child's *present level* of movement pattern development and should indicate the *level to be achieved* by the child.

While attempting to improve motor skills, the motor development specialist may also contribute to cognitive and affective growth through movement activities. The instructor should formulate specific objectives for each of the five basic movement patterns. Figure 5–3 lists the two types of movement abilities and the physical abilities necessary for successful performance.

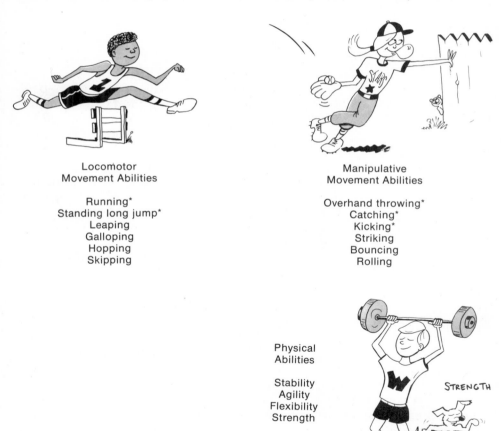

Locomotor
Movement Abilities

Running*
Standing long jump*
Leaping
Galloping
Hopping
Skipping

Manipulative
Movement Abilities

Overhand throwing*
Catching*
Kicking*
Striking
Bouncing
Rolling

Physical
Abilities

Stability
Agility
Flexibility
Strength

STRENGTH

Figure 5–3 The abilities essential to efficient fundamental movement. (The asterisk indicates the basic movement patterns.)

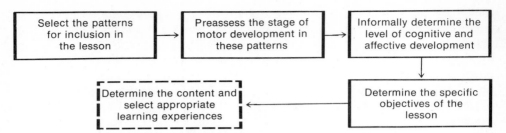

Figure 5–4   Determining the specific objectives and learning experiences for inclusion in the motor development program.

When developing specific objectives for the lesson, the instructor first needs to select the patterns to be worked on. Then he must determine the child's or group's stage of motor development in that particular pattern and the appropriate learning level of the child or children involved. Figure 5–4 is a visual representation of the steps involved in ascertaining the specific objectives of the program.

DETERMINE APPROPRIATE LEARNING EXPERIENCES

Once the specific objectives of the lesson and program have been decided upon, it becomes an easy matter of selecting the learning experiences to be included in the lesson. We have already determined the child's present level of motor development and the level we expect the child to achieve. The question to be asked now is, *"How can we help him achieve that level?"* The answer lies in structuring specific movement experiences geared toward this end. The movement activities may take many forms and may be presented to the learner through a wide variety of teaching techniques or styles. It is not within the scope of this text to provide a detailed discussion of teacher behavior. However, the reader is referred to Chapter 8 for a brief discussion of common teaching styles appropriate for use in either the developmental or the remedial fundamental movement program.

The specific learning experiences in the lesson should help children develop their *fundamental movement abilities* and their *physical abilities.* Activities for working on fundamental movement abilities should improve specific *locomotor* and *manipulative* patterns. Movement activities should also enhance the physical qualities of *stability, agility, flexibility,* and *strength,* which are essential for efficient pattern development and refinement.

The manner in which we structure and present the movement activities to be included in the lesson can also help us influence the child's cognitive and affective development. It must be remembered that the chief goal of the movement pattern program advocated in this text is helping children learn to move more efficiently by improving their psychomotor functioning. It is *through* achievement of this primary aim that we, as concerned and skilled teachers, can also make important contributions to the child's cognitive and affective behavior. For example, movement experiences may affect *cognitive development* by promoting *academic concept development* and *perceptual-motor efficiency.* Further, they may contribute to *affective development* by improving *self concept, peer relations,* and *play skills.*

The movement experiences contained in Chapters 9 to 11 are intended to serve only as examples of how one may develop and implement a series of activities that will satisfy the child's developmental and remedial needs.

POST-PROGRAM ASSESSMENT

The final step in the process of curriculum planning, no less important than the preceding steps, involves frequent reassessment of the child's level of development. Reassessment of the developmental level is crucial, for only in this way can we be certain that the specific objectives and specially planned learning experiences are appropriate for the child. If over a period of time the learning experiences are successful in helping the child achieve the specific objectives set up by the instructor, then those selected experiences have been appropriate. The child should now be exposed to general movement activities that include participation in modified versions of sports (lead-up games) and development of sport skills. If the child does not acquire mature patterns of movement, the instructor must attempt to structure new learning experiences that will be successful in helping the child do so.

Reassessment of a young child usually does not involve formal skill testing, since individuals familiar with the progressive acquisition of movement and the techniques of observing movement can readily determine whether a child has reached a mature level of functioning. The observational technique outlined in Chapter 6 enables the motor development specialist to assess the child's progress informally on a continual basis. This constant monitoring of movement enables the teacher to structure developmentally appropriate movement experiences throughout the duration of the program.

SUMMARY

The initial step in designing and implementing a motor development program is establishment of the aims and general objectives of the program. The aims include helping the child learn to move and assisting him to learn through movement. The general objectives are developmental and remedial; the decision whether to use one or both objectives depends upon the needs of the children involved in the program.

In order to design an appropriate program for the improvement of fundamental movement patterns, we must determine the developmental level of the children involved. This means assessing their level of cognitive and affective development as well as their level of psychomotor functioning.

Once this has been accomplished, we can determine the specific objectives of the program. Although these objectives are primarily psychomotor,

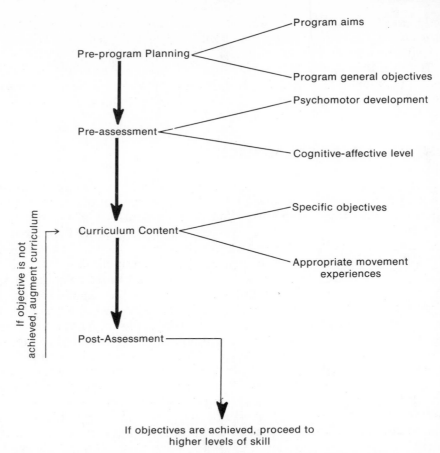

Figure 5–5   A curricular model for developing a program designed to enhance fundamental movement patterns.

cognitive and affective objectives may also be achieved through psychomotor activities. The next step in the process is to decide which movement activities best promote specific movement and physical abilities. The final step in the program is to evaluate the children's progress and make appropriate changes to meet their needs. Figure 5–5 is a visual representation of the program model outlined in this chapter.

BIBLIOGRAPHY

1. Bloom, Benjamin (ed.): *Taxonomy of Educational Objectives.* New York: David McKay, 1956.
2. Buros, Oscar K.: *Mental Measurements Yearbook,* 2 vols. 7th ed. Highland Park, N. J.: Gryphon Press, 1972.
3. Erikson, Erik: *Childhood and Society.* New York: Norton, 1963.
4. Espenschade, Anna S., and Eckert, Helen M.: *Motor Development.* Columbus, Ohio: Charles E. Merrill, 1967, p. 106.

5. Gessell, Arnold: *The First Five Years of Life: A Guide to the Study of the Preschool Child.* New York: Harper and Brothers, 1940.
6. Godfrey, Barbara B., and Kephart, Newell C.: *Movement Patterns and Motor Education.* New York: Appleton-Century-Crofts, 1969.
7. Mager, Robert F.: *Preparing Instructional Objectives.* Palo Alto, Calif.: Fearon Publishers, 1962.
8. Piaget, Jean: *The Origins of Intelligence in Children.* New York: International Universities Press, 1952.
9. Rarick, G. Lawrence: *Motor Development During Infancy and Early Childhood.* Madison, Wisc.: College Printing and Typing Co. 1961, p. 48.
10. Sinclair, Caroline B.: *Movement of the Young Child: Ages Two to Six.* Columbus, Ohio: Charles E. Merrill, 1972.

CHAPTER 6

OBSERVING AND EVALUATING FUNDAMENTAL MOVEMENT PATTERNS

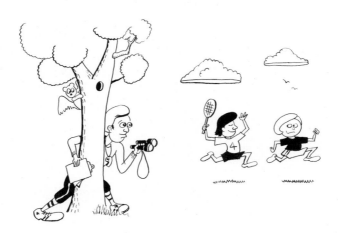

Teachers and parents concerned with the motor development of young or poorly coordinated children should be interested in the *quality* as well as *quantity* of human movement. Unfortunately, current performance-based measurement techniques, emphasizing quantity of movement, are limited in their ability to identify particular developmental weaknesses in the fundamental movement patterns of young children. Poor performance is often attributed to lack of strength or coordination when, in fact, it may be due to a developmental lag in the acquisition of the mature movement pattern.

For many years physical educators and other professionals have used assessment techniques to evaluate physical fitness, motor ability, and skill proficiency. These quantitative measures often are of limited value, however, in attempts to evaluate the motor development of the young or poorly coordinated child. Some educators have been overly concerned with the child's ability to perform a motor skill at some predetermined level. Although this approach does identify children who exhibit inefficient body movement, it does not isolate specifically what is wrong with the movement.

Qualitative assessment of fundamental movement patterns, on the other hand, enables the teacher to identify specific weaknesses in a specific pattern. It indicates the quality of the movement performed in relation to the mature pattern. Although of greater value to the elementary educator, qualitative assessment techniques in the past generally have not been administratively feasible for extensive school use.

An observation technique for evaluating fundamental movement patterns has been developed for use with young and poorly coordinated children. With this method of qualitative assessment, several children may be observed and evaluated in a relatively short period of time. Children who are delayed in acquiring fundamental movement abilities may be singled out and offered appropriate movement activities to enhance their motor development. Early identification of these children facilitates the improvement of inefficient movements. Children who have acquired mature patterns can be offered activities designed to increase their performance level or can begin incorporating these fundamental patterns into more advanced sport or game skills.

The following observational technique, constructed from current available literature and research on the development of fundamental movement patterns during early childhood, has been designed to satisfy the following objectives:

1. To develop a technique that will subjectively evaluate the development of children's fundamental movement patterns, so that this information may be utilized as a reliable pre-program or post-program evaluation of children participating in a motor development program.
2. To develop a technique to identify children experiencing difficulty with fundamental movements, so that these children may be offered additional opportunities for improvement.
3. To perpetuate, through use of the technique, an awareness in motor development specialists, physical educators, regular classroom teachers, and special education teachers of the sequence of acquisition of movement abilities during childhood and the body mechanics involved.

SELECTION OF THE MOVEMENT PATTERNS

A movement pattern consists of a series of body actions that combine to form an integrated act involving the whole body. Five movement patterns have been selected for subjective evaluation by this observational technique. These patterns include: (1) running a short distance for speed; (2) jumping for horizontal distance with both feet; (3) throwing a ball for distance in an overhand manner; (4) catching a small ball tossed at chest height; and (5) kicking a ball for distance with one lead-in step. In the selection of the movement patterns to be evaluated, the following considerations were taken into account.

The patterns selected should represent movements that are essential for more sophisticated motor skill development. The movement patterns to be evaluated form the foundation on which more complex movement and sport skills are based. Young children experiencing difficulty in acquiring efficient fundamental movements later often have difficulty performing more complex skills. Evaluation, therefore, identifies children at an early age who may have difficulty with later, more advanced motor skills.

The patterns selected included movements that children utilize daily in their normal play activities. The patterns to be evaluated should be familiar to the child, since performance of an untypical motor skill would not give the evaluator an accurate picture of the child's level of motor development. Movement patterns are improved with experience; therefore, the child must be familiar with the movement to be evaluated. For example, adults throwing a ball with their nondominant hand exhibit an immature pattern. Performance of this untypical movement thus does not give a valid indication of the individual's level of movement refinement. In addition to insuring an accurate assessment, selecting movement patterns performed during normal play activity allows the evaluator to collect informal data continually throughout the course of the child's development.

The patterns selected should be similar to movements that have been or could be easily measured by objective, performance-based testing. In some instances it may be desirable to obtain both qualitative and quantitative information on a child. Similar patterns must be measured so that the results may be validly compared. This information enables the evaluator to compare the child's performance to norms and to identify developmental lags in the acquisition of the mature movement pattern. Moreover, a comparison of the two results showing that performance is low but that the movement exhibited resembles the mature pattern may indicate weakness in a pattern component, such as strength, coordination, or flexibility.

The quality of a child's movement must be evaluated by comparison with some standard. In performance, or quantitative, measures, this standard usually consists of well-established norms. Qualitative evaluation must use some similar basis for comparison in order to determine a child's motor weaknesses.

Research on the patterns selected must be sufficiently complete to ascertain whether there are developmental trends in the acquisition of the mature movement pattern. Enough studies have been conducted on children throughout the early childhood period (2 to 6 years of age) to identify specific developmental changes that occur in the refinement of several movement patterns. Once identified, these trends may be used to establish a developmental progression for each of the patterns. Movement patterns lacking sufficient research data for construction of a developmental progression were not selected for evaluation by the technique outlined in this text.

CONSTRUCTION OF A DEVELOPMENTAL PROGRESSION

Specific trends in the development of fundamental movements have been identified and a developmental progression established for each pattern. This progression, divided into the three stages of motor development during the early childhood period, is presented in Table 6–1.

Ages have deliberately not been assigned to the developmental stages because of the various rates at which children refine fundamental movements. Individual rates of maturation and varying environment conditions may either speed up or slow down development. Children beyond the age of 7 years who have not achieved mature movement patterns should be offered a remedial or enrichment program of physical activities to improve their motor development. This prevents children from passing through the critical period of early childhood without developing fundamental movement patterns to their maximum potential.

Table 6–1 DEVELOPMENTAL STAGES OF EARLY CHILDHOOD

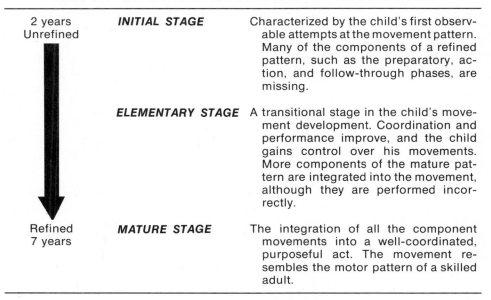

2 years Unrefined	*INITIAL STAGE*	Characterized by the child's first observable attempts at the movement pattern. Many of the components of a refined pattern, such as the preparatory, action, and follow-through phases, are missing.
	ELEMENTARY STAGE	A transitional stage in the child's movement development. Coordination and performance improve, and the child gains control over his movements. More components of the mature pattern are integrated into the movement, although they are performed incorrectly.
Refined 7 years	*MATURE STAGE*	The integration of all the component movements into a well-coordinated, purposeful act. The movement resembles the motor pattern of a skilled adult.

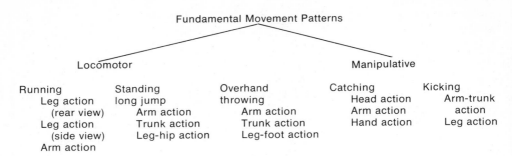

Figure 6–1   Body actions of the selected locomotor and manipulative fundamental movement patterns.

To help the observer utilize the observational technique, each of the five selected movement patterns has been divided into three (two for kicking) body actions (Fig. 6–1). The evaluator can thus concentrate on observing the action of one body part.

In order for each body action of the movement to be evaluated individually, the child should perform each pattern a minimum of three times (two for kicking). In some instances, it may be necessary to observe the child more than three times to obtain a valid judgment. The only limit on the number of performances by a child is his ability to give valid representations of his skill in performing the act. It is therefore recommended that the child, because of possible fatigue and boredom, attempt only three trials of a particular pattern in a formal observational setting. Informal observations may continue, however, as long as the child retains interest in performing and does not tire. Evaluations may be completed after a short period of time or during the next few days.

The following pages contain directions for using the observational technique. The developmental progresssions for each of the selected movement patterns are visually as well as textually presented to help the observer familiarize himself with the changes that occur in the refinement of the selected movements. On the evaluation sheet, key phrases from the developmental progressions help the observer recall the patterns at the three stages of development.

OBSERVATIONAL TECHNIQUE FOR EVALUATING FUNDAMENTAL MOVEMENT PATTERNS

The technique for evaluating selected fundamental movement patterns may be utilized in whole (all the patterns) or in part (selected individual patterns), depending upon the information desired. In addition, this technique may permit the observer to evaluate the movement patterns of a single child or a class of children either formally or informally.

Children may be observed informally during a regular physical education class or during normal play activities on the playground. After watching the child, the evaluator should note the child's performance on a summary sheet. Formal observation normally takes place in a structured setting on a one-to-one basis. It is recommended that those unfamiliar with observing fundamental movement attempt several formal observations in order to develop sufficient skill to evaluate movement accurately in an informal setting.

To insure that each child being observed is performing a pattern similar to the movements in the text, it is important to consider the following points.

Children who are being observed must perform the movement to the best of their ability. This often can be accomplished by verbal instructions like "as far as you can" or "as hard as you can." Care must be taken, however, not to force children to do what they cannot because they tend to revert to a less mature level of functioning when performing beyond their ability. It must also be borne in mind that children often use a different pattern as the objective of the movement changes. For example, the mature pattern for throwing a dart accurately is similar to the elementary stage of the overhand throw for distance.

Whenever possible, children should not be made aware that they are being observed. An observer with a clipboard standing right next to a child may inhibit the child and lower his performance level. The observer should be sufficiently aware of the key actions to evaluate a total pattern before actually recording any results. If possible, one instructor may play with the child and structure the play around the pattern to be studied while a second observer records the results.

Young children have a short interest span; therefore, it may be necessary to observe the movement patterns on various days. Since each movement pattern should be performed three or more times, it is vital that the children enjoy performing. Observations should not be continued if the child indicates that he or she is bored. Verbal praise and assuring physical contact reinforce the performance. In some instances, the specific movement may be incorporated into a game to increase the child's interest.

The child should, when possible, be given only a verbal description of the pattern to be performed. If a child is unable to perform the movement correctly on the basis of the verbal description, he should be put through the movement manually. A movement should be demonstrated only when the child cannot produce the pattern after being told about the movement and helped to perform it. Demonstrating a pattern may give the child cues to the mature movement and therefore result in an invalid observation.

The observational technique for evaluating fundamental movement patterns in young or poorly coordinated children is presented in three sections: (1) Developmental Progressions of the Selected Patterns, (2) Movement Pattern Evaluation sheets, and (3) Information Summary sheets.

The *Developmental Progressions of the Selected Patterns* have each been divided into an initial, elementary, and mature stage based on information from available research literature. In addition, each of these developmental progressions has been further divided into observable body actions. The observer should learn about each stage in the acquisition of a particular pattern and the refinements in body action that take place with maturity.

To help the instructor identify the developmental changes that take place, pictorial representations of the movements have been included with each developmental progression. These pictures have been drawn from motion picture film of right- and left-handed children performing the selected patterns.

In learning about children's movement, the observer may find it helpful to supplement study of the developmental progressions with observations of young children in the gymnasium or on the playground. The authors have found the use of Super 8 film, taken at 48 frames per second and shown through a projector with "step" (single frame) motion, to be invaluable for rapidly sharpening observation skills.

Once totally familiar with the developmental progressions of the selected patterns, the instructor is ready to use observation in evaluating a child's performance. *Movement Pattern Evaluation sheets,* to be used for individual evaluation, have been developed to help the observer remember the specific actions and refinements to be assessed.

The upper portion of each individual evaluation sheet contains information the observer may find useful, including (1) the recommended observation position, (2) special instructions for the particular pattern, (3) suggested verbal directions, and (4) a space for the performer's name and birthdate. On the lower portion of each sheet is a checklist that summarizes the developmental progressions and, by using key phrases, helps the observer to recall trends in pattern refinement. The description of each particular body action is arranged horizontally on the sheet, proceeding in order from the initial to the mature stage.

Keeping in mind the instructions given initially in this section, the observer assumes the recommended observing position and instructs the child to perform. The observer should attempt to evaluate only one body action per performance. Determine which stage best typifies the action performed and check the appropriate box. Particular strengths and weaknesses may also be noted by checking any applicable key phrases within a particular stage of an action. Further comments may be made in the appropriate space below each series of key phrases.

The information from the individual evaluation sheets may be compiled by using the *Information Summary sheets* found in the third seciton. Data may be easily transferred from each performer's individual evaluation sheets to the Class Information summary and the Class Ability chart. The instructor is now supplied with the information about quality of movement that is needed for designing and planning appropriate movement experiences to satisfy the developmental needs of the class or individual child.

DEVELOPMENTAL PROGRESSIONS OF
THE SELECTED PATTERNS

DIRECTIONS:

1. Identify those patterns that are to be evaluated.
2. Study the developmental progressions of the patterns to be observed.
3. Identify specific developmental changes that take place as each action for a particular pattern is refined. (Example: leg-foot actions of the throwing pattern may progress from *no step*, to *a step on the same side* as the throwing arm and finally to *a step in opposition* to the throwing motion.)

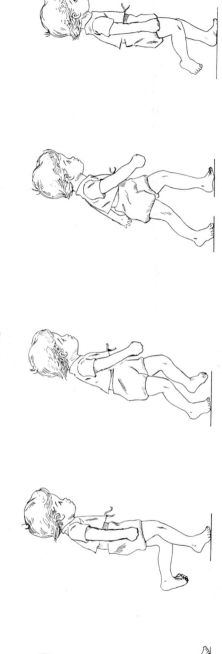

RUNNING

Initial Stage

Leg Action (Side View)

The legs appear stiff and the stride is uneven. There is no observable flight phase, and the base of support is wide. The swing of the leg is short and limited.

Leg Action (Rear View)

The recovery knee is swung outward, then around and forward to a support position. The swinging foot tends to rotate outward from the hip, which allows the foot to be swung forward without a great deal of body lift and thereby helps the child to maintain balance.

Arm Action

The arms swing stiffly with varying degrees of flexion at the elbow. The range of motion of the arms is short, as the arms tend to swing outward horizontally rather than vertically. This outward rotation counteracts the excessive rotary movement of the swinging leg.

RUNNING

Elementary Stage

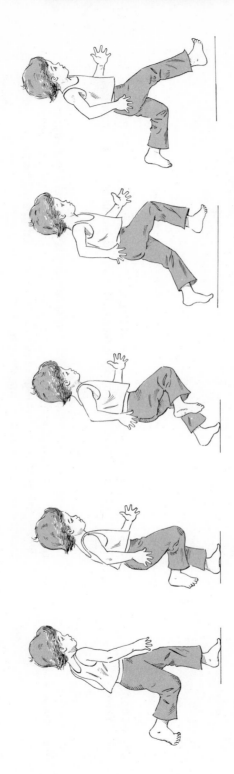

Leg Action (Side View)

Stride length, leg swing, and speed increase. There is a definite observable flight phase to the pattern. The support leg begins to extend more completely at takeoff.

Leg Action (Rear View)

At the height of recovery to the rear, the recovery foot swings across the midline before it is swung forward to the contact position.

Arm Action

The arms swing for a greater distance vertically, and there is limited horizontal movement on the backswing as the child's stride length increases.

RUNNING

Mature Stage

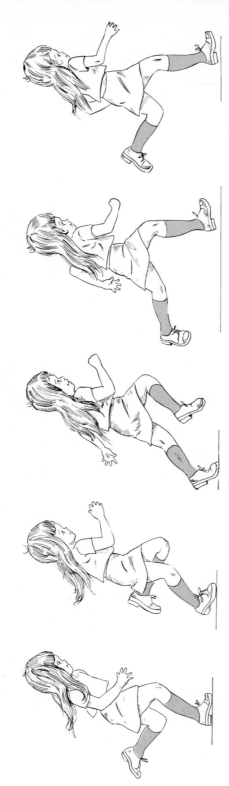

Leg Action (Side View)

The recovery knee is raised high and swung forward quickly. The support leg bends slightly at contact and then extends completely and quickly through the hip, knee, and ankle. The length of the stride and the duration of flight time are at their maximum.

Leg Action (Rear View)

There is very little rotary action of the recovery knee or foot as the length of the stride increases.

Arm Action

The arms swing vertically in a large arc in opposition to the legs. The arms are bent at the elbows in approximate right angles.

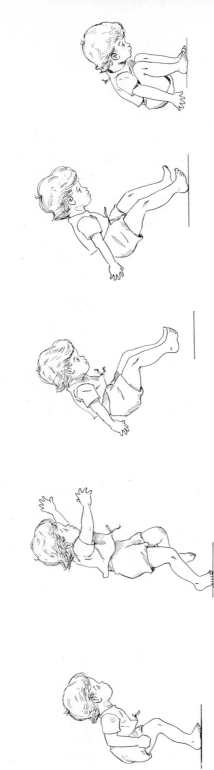

JUMPING

Initial Stage

Arm Action

The arms, limited in their swing, do not initiate the jumping action. They move in a sideward-downward or rearward-upward direction to maintain balance during the flight.

Trunk Action

The trunk at takeoff is propelled in a vertical direction with little emphasis upon the length of the jump.

Leg-Hip Action

The preparatory crouch is limited and inconsistent with regard to the degree of leg flexion. At takeoff and landing the child has difficulty using both feet simultaneously, and one leg may precede the other. The extension of the hips, legs, and ankles is incomplete at the takeoff of the jump.

JUMPING

Elementary Stage

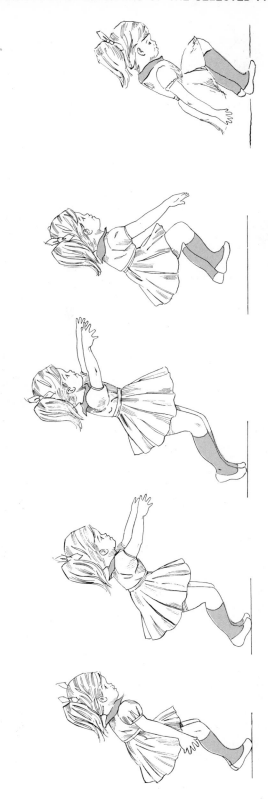

Arm Action

The arms are utilized more productively in the jumping action. They initiate the pattern at takeoff and then move to the side to maintain balance during the jump.

Trunk Action

No observable change.

Leg-Hip Action

The preparatory crouch is deeper and more consistent. The legs, hips, and ankles extend more at takeoff; however, they remain somewhat bent. During the flight, the thighs are held in a flexed position.

JUMPING

Mature Stage

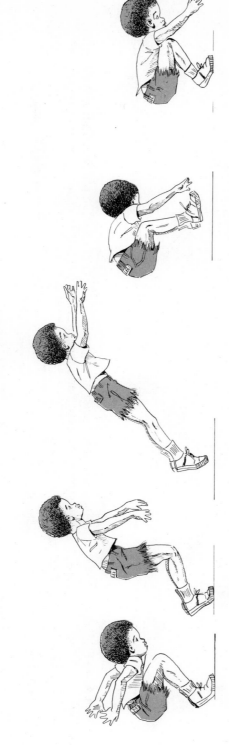

Arm Action

The arms move high and to the rear and then reach forward during the take-off. The arms are held high throughout the jumping action.

Trunk Action

The trunk at takeoff is propelled at an angle of approximately 45 degrees. The major emphasis is on the horizontal direction of the jump.

Leg-Hip Action

The preparatory crouch is deep and consistent. The hips, legs, and ankles are completely extended at takeoff. During the flight, the hips flex, bringing the thighs to a position nearly horizontal to the ground. The lower leg hangs in a nearly-vertical position. The body weight upon landing continues forward and downward.

THROWING

Initial Stage

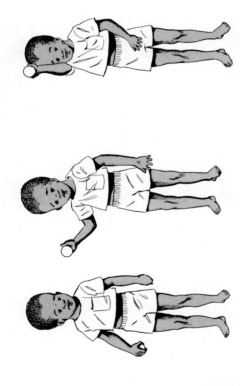

Arm Action

The throwing motion is performed mainly from the elbow, which remains in front of the body. The throw consists of a pushing action. At the point of release, the fingers are spread. The follow-through is forward and downward.

Trunk Action

The trunk remains perpendicular to the target throughout the throw. There is very little shoulder rotation during the throwing motion. The child tends to move slightly backward as the throw is made.

Leg-Foot Action

The feet remain stationary, although there may be some purposeless shifting of the feet during preparation for the throw.

THROWING

Elementary Stage

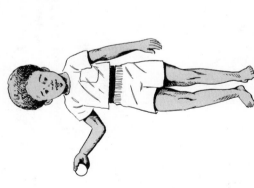

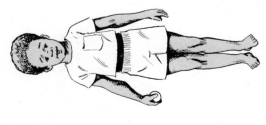

Arm Action

The arm is swung in preparation, first sideward-upward and then backward to a position of elbow flexion where the ball is brought to a position behind the head. The arm swings forward in a high over-the-shoulder action. The follow-through is forward and downward. The wrist completes the throw, and the ball is controlled more by the fingers.

Trunk Action

The trunk rotates toward the throwing side during the preparatory phase of the throw. As the arm initiates the throwing action, the trunk rotates back toward the nonthrowing side. The trunk flexes forward with the forward motion of the throwing arm.

Leg-Foot Action

The performer steps forward with the leg that is on the same side as the throwing arm. There is a forward shift in the body weight.

THROWING
Mature Stage

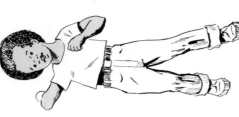
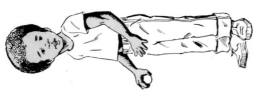
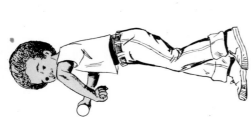
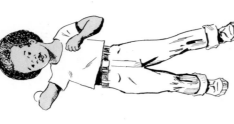
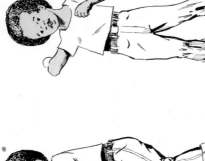

Arm Action

The arm swings backward in preparation for the throw. The throwing elbow moves forward horizontally as it extends. The thumb rotates in and downward and therefore ends up pointing downward. At release the fingers remain close together.

Trunk Action

During the preparatory phase of the throw, the trunk is markedly rotated to the throwing side and the throwing shoulder drops slightly. As the forward motion begins, the trunk rotates through the hips, spine, and shoulders. The throwing shoulder rotates to a position in line with the target.

Leg-Foot Action

During the preparatory phase of the throw, the weight is on the rear foot. As the trunk rotates, the weight is completely shifted with a step on the foot that is on the nonthrowing side of the body.

CATCHING
Initial Stage

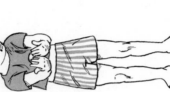
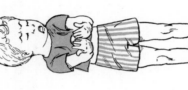
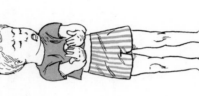
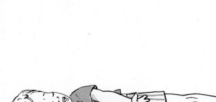
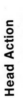
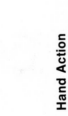

Head Action

As the ball is thrown, there is a definite avoidance reaction of turning the face away from the thrown ball or protecting the head with the arms and hands.

Arm Action

The arms are held out with the elbows extended in front of the body. There is limited arm movement until contact with the ball is made. The catching pattern resembles a scooping action as the performer attempts to direct the ball to the chest. The catch is poorly timed.

Hand Action

The fingers are extended and held tense. There is very little use of the hands during this stage of the catching pattern.

CATCHING

Elementary Stage

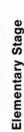
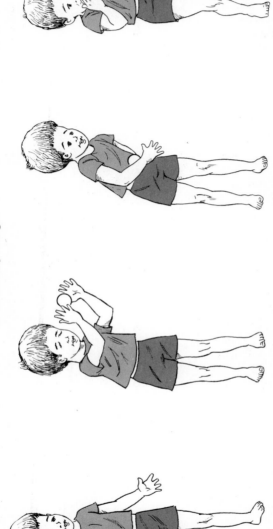

Head Action

The performer exhibits an avoidance reaction only by closing the eyes when contact with the ball is made.

Arm Action

The arms are held slightly bent in front of the body. The performer attempts initial contact with the hands; however, timing is poor and the ball is then clasped to the body with the arms.

Hand Action

The hands are held in opposition to each other in preparation for the throw. The fingers are extended and begin to point increasingly toward the ball in anticipation of the catch. As contact is made with the ball, the hands close unevenly in a poorly timed motion.

CATCHING

Mature Stage

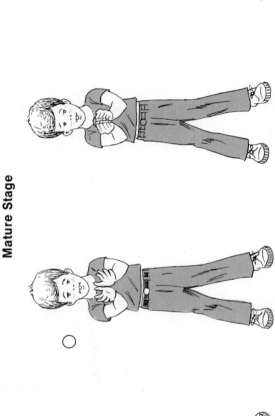

Head Action   The avoidance reaction has been completely suppressed. The eyes follow the ball from the point of release to final contact.

Arm Action   The arms are bent at the elbows and held relaxed at the sides or in front of the body in preparation for the throw. The arms give upon contact with the ball to absorb its force. The arms make adjustments to variations (changes in height, for example) in the flight of the ball.

Hand Action   The hands are cupped together with either the thumbs or the little fingers in opposition, depending upon the height of the tossed ball. In a well-timed motion, the hands are clasped together as contact is made.

KICKING

Initial Stage

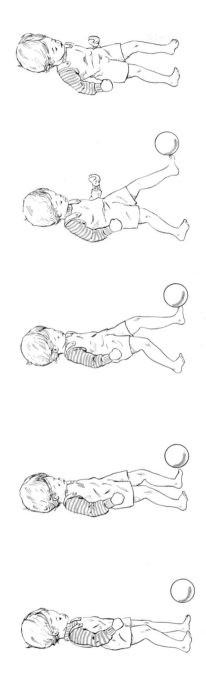

Arm-Trunk Action

The movement of the arms and trunk is limited during the kicking action. The body remains erect, with the arms held down at the sides or out for stability.

Leg Action

The kicking leg is limited to the backswing during the preparatory phase of the kick. The forward swing is short, and there is no follow-through. Rather than kicking the ball squarely, the leg tends to kick "at" the ball.

KICKING

Elementary Stage

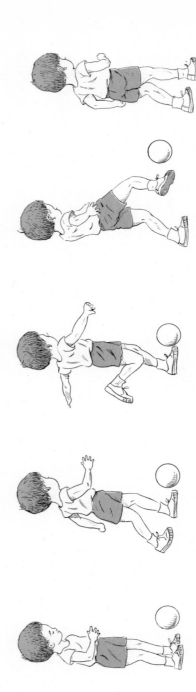

Arm-Trunk Action

No observable change.

Leg Action

The kicking leg is brought backward during the preparatory phase of the kick, which is made from the knee. The kicking leg tends to remain bent until the ball has been contacted.

KICKING

Mature Stage

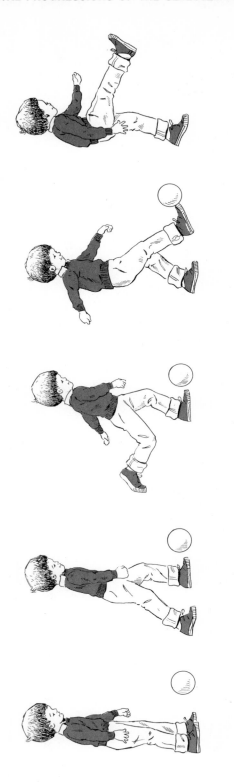

Arm-Trunk Action

As contact is made with the ball, the arm on the kicking side tends to swing from a forward to a backward position while the other arm tends to move from a backward or sideward position to a forward one. The trunk bends at the waist during the follow-through.

Leg Action

The movement of the kicking leg is initiated at the hip, and there is limited knee bend. The leg swings through a long arc, and the support leg bends upon contact with the ball. During the follow-through, the support foot raises to its toes. The foot kicks with a complete and high follow-through.

MOVEMENT PATTERN EVALUATION SHEETS

DIRECTIONS:

1. Become totally familiar with the developmental progression for each pattern to be observed.
2. Study the individual evaluation sheet for each pattern to be observed.
3. Decide whether the observation will take place in a formal or informal setting.
4. Become familiar with the correct observation position, suggested verbal directions, and special instructions for each pattern.
5. Station yourself in the proper observation position and instruct the child to perform the pattern a minimum of three times (two for kicking).
6. Observe only one action on each attempt. Identify the stage of development that best describes the child's performance and check (✔) that box.
7. Specific areas of weakness in an action may be noted by placing a slash (/) in the appropriate blank across from key phrases.
8. Observe each action separately until all actions have been evaluated. Make any additional comments on the back of each evaluation sheet.

NAME _____
BIRTHDATE _____

RUNNING

Observation Position: The running pattern should be observed from two different locations. Leg action (side view) and arm action should be assessed from the side of the performer at a distance of approximately 20 feet, whereas leg action (rear view) should be observed from behind the performer as he runs away from the observer. The performer should start and finish on a clearly marked line. It may be helpful to place the child in a competitive situation to encourage him to exert maximum effort. The running distance should be long enough for the child to reach maximum speed; however, the child should not be fatigued. A sufficient rest period must be given between trials.

Suggested Verbal Directions: "When I say *go*, I want you to run as fast as you can to those _____ (cones, chairs, and so on). Ready? Go."

Special Instructions: When determining the length of the run, the instructor must consider:
(1) Having sufficient time to evaluate the action to be observed (not counting the initial acceleration and final deceleration phases of the run).
(2) The age of the child and the ability of the child to perform the run without tiring during any attempt. It is suggested that for children under 6 years of age the total distance be limited to under 15 to 20 yards; older children may attempt from 25 to 35 yards. The running surface should be level and smooth; rough ground may alter the pattern exhibited.

	INITIAL	ELEMENTARY	MATURE
LEG ACTION (Side View)	☐ — Leg swing is short, limited — Stiff, uneven stride — No observable flight phase — Incomplete extension of support leg	☐ — Length, swing, and speed increase — Limited but observable flight phase — Support leg extends more completely at takeoff	☐ — Length of stride is at its maximum; speed of stride is fast — Definite flight phase — Support leg extends completely — Recovery thigh is parallel to ground
ARM ACTION	☐ — Stiff, short swing; varying degrees of elbow flexion — Tend to swing outward horizontally	☐ — Arm swing increases — Horizontal swing is reduced on backswing	☐ — Swing vertically in opposition to the legs — Arms are bent in approximate right angles
LEG ACTION (Rear View)	☐ — Swinging leg rotates outward from the hip — Swinging foot toes outward — Wide base of support	☐ — Swinging foot crosses midline at height of recovery to rear	☐ — Little rotary action of recovery leg and foot

103

STANDING LONG JUMP

NAME

BIRTHDATE

Observation Position: The standing long jump should be observed from a position perpendicular to the action. The performer should start in a relaxed position with toes of both feet touching the starting line. Care should be taken not to place the child's feet in an uncomfortable starting position.

Suggested Verbal Directions: "When I tell you to jump, I want you to jump with *both* feet as far as you can. Ready? Jump."

Special Instructions: The standing long jump pattern should be performed on a mat or a soft, grassy surface. The starting position should be marked with a line; footprints cut from paper may help the child place his feet in the appropriate position.

	INITIAL	ELEMENTARY	MATURE
ARM ACTION	— Limited swing; arms do not initiate jumping action — During flight, sideward-downward or rearward upward action to maintain balance	— Initiate jumping action — Always remain toward front of body during preparatory crouch — Move out to side to maintain balance during flight.	— Move high and to the rear during preparatory crouch — During takeoff, they swing forward with force and reach high — Arms are held high throughout the jumping action
TRUNK ACTION	— Moves in vertical direction; little emphasis upon length of jump		— Trunk is propelled at approximately a 45-degree angle — Major emphasis is on horizontal distance
LEG-HIP ACTION	— Preparatory crouch is inconsistent in terms of leg flexion — Difficulty using both feet — Extension at takeoff is limited — Weight falls backward at landing	— Preparatory crouch is deeper and more consistent — Extension is more complete at takeoff — Hips are flexed during flight, and thighs are held in a flexed position	— Preparatory crouch is deep and consistent — Complete extension of ankles, knees, and hips at takeoff — Thighs are held parallel to ground during flight; lower leg hangs vertically — Body weight at landing is forward

OVERHAND THROWING

NAME _____
BIRTHDATE _____

Observation Position: The overhand throwing pattern should be observed while the evaluator is directly facing the performer and standing slightly off center on the child's dominant side. Care should be taken not to obstruct or limit the child's throw by blocking the direction of the throw.

Suggested Verbal Directions: "When I tell you, I want you to throw this ball as far as you can. Ready? Throw."

Special Instructions: The throwing surface should be level and not slippery. If possible, the pattern should be performed outside or in a large gymnasium. The ball should be small enough so the child can easily control it with the fingers. Wiffle balls are excellent because they can be thrown only limited distances and therefore can be easily retrieved.

	INITIAL	ELEMENTARY	MATURE
ARM ACTION	☐ Motion is mainly from elbow — Elbow remains in front of body; action resembles push — Fingers spread at release — Follow-through is forward and downward	☐ In preparation arm is swung upward, sideward and backward to position of elbow flexion — Ball is held behind head — Arm is swung forward, high over the shoulder	☐ Arm is swung backward in preparation — Opposite elbow is raised to balance preparatory action in throwing arm — Throwing elbow moves forward horizontally as it extends — Forearm rotates and thumb ends up pointing downward
TRUNK ACTION	☐ Trunk remains perpendicular to target — Little rotary action during throw — Body weight shifts slightly rearward	☐ Trunk rotates toward throwing side during preparatory action — Shoulders rotate toward throwing side — Trunk flexes forward with forward motion of arm — Definite forward shift of body weight	☐ Trunk markedly rotates to throwing side during preparatory action — Throwing shoulder drops slightly — A definite rotation through hips, legs, spine, and shoulders during throw
LEG-FOOT ACTION	☐ Feet remain stationary — Purposeless shifting of feet during preparation of throw	☐ Steps forward with leg on same side as throwing arm	☐ Weight during preparatory movement is on rear foot — As weight is shifted, there is a step with the opposite foot

CATCHING

NAME
BIRTHDATE

Observation Position: The catching pattern should be observed while the observer stands directly in front of the performer and faces him. Using an underhand pitch, the observer should toss a small ball to the child at approximately chest height.

Suggested Verbal Directions: "I want you to catch this ball when I throw it to you. Ready?"

Special Instructions: The size and weight of the ball is an important factor in the catching pattern exhibited by the young child. It is recommended that the observer use a softball-sized Wiffle or fluff ball. The height of the tossed ball will also alter the exhibited pattern. The ball should be tossed at approximately chest height from a distance of 5 feet. Any toss too low or too high should be disregarded.

INITIAL STAGE

HEAD ACTION

☐ — Definite avoidance reaction of turning face away or protecting face with arms

ARM ACTION

☐ — Arms are extended and held in front of body
— Limited movement until contact
— Action resembles scooping action
— Attempts to use body to trap ball

HAND ACTION

☐ — Palms are held upward
— Fingers are extended and held tense
— Hands are not utilized in the catching action

ELEMENTARY STAGE

☐ — Avoidance reaction is limited to the child's closing the eyes at contact with ball

☐ — Elbows are held at sides with approximately 90-degree bend
— Since initial contact made with the child's hands is often unsuccessful, the arms trap ball

☐ — Hands are held in opposition to each other; thumbs are held upward
— At contact the hands attempt to squeeze the ball in a poorly timed and uneven motion

MATURE STAGE

☐ — Avoidance reaction is completely suppressed

☐ — Arms are held relaxed at sides, and forearms are held in front of body
— Arms give upon contact to absorb force of ball
— Arms adjust to flight of ball

☐ — Thumbs are held in opposition to each other
— Hands grasp ball in a well-timed, simultaneous motion
— Fingers make a more effective grasping motion

NAME _____
BIRTHDATE _____

KICKING

Observation Position: The kicking pattern should be observed from the side of the performer, with the observer standing directly perpendicular to the ball that is to be kicked.

Suggested Verbal Directions: "When I tell you, I want you to kick this ball as hard and as far as you can. Ready? Kick."

Special Instructions: The child should be placed in a position approximately one step away from the ball. The kick should not be made from a running start. The ball should be approximately 10 to 12 inches in diameter and not hard enough to inhibit the kicking action.

INITIAL

ARM-TRUNK ACTION

☐
— Movements are restricted during the kicking action
— Trunk remains erect
— Arms are used to maintain balance

LEG ACTION

☐
— Kicking leg is limited in backswing
— Forward swing is short; no follow-through
— Child kicks "at" ball rather than kicking it squarely and following through

ELEMENTARY

☐
— Preparatory backswing is centered at knee
— Kicking leg tends to remain bent throughout kick
— Follow-through is limited to forward movement of knee

MATURE

☐
— Arms swing in opposition to each other during kicking action
— Trunk bends at waist during follow-through

☐
— Movement of kicking leg is initiated at hip
— Support leg bends slightly at contact
— Length of leg swing increases
— Follow-through is high; support foot rises to its toes

INFORMATION SUMMARY SHEETS

DIRECTIONS:

If a group or class of children is to be observed and the instructor is concerned with identifying class strengths and weaknesses:
1. Complete the Class Information Summary sheet by summarizing information from individual evaluation sheets.
2. Graph the totals from the Class Information Summary sheet on the Class Ability chart.
3. Identify the strengths and weaknesses of the class in the appropriate section of the Class Information Summary sheet.
4. Provide class with age-appropriate movement experiences to improve motor abilities.

If a single child or a group of children is to be observed and the instructor wants to identify strengths and weaknesses of individual children:
1. Summarize information from the child's individual evaluation sheets.
2. Complete an Individual Profile chart on each child.
3. Identify the various strengths and weaknesses of a child's performance.
4. Provide the child with age-appropriate activities to improve motor abilities.

CLASS SUMMARY SHEET

DATE

TOTALS

NAME

| | I E M | I E M | I E M | I E M | I E M | I E M | I E M | I E M | I E M | I E M | I E M | | I E M |

RUNNING
 Leg action (side)
 Arm action
 Leg action (rear)
JUMPING
 Arm action
 Trunk action
 Leg-hip action
THROWING
 Arm action
 Trunk action
 Leg-foot action
CATCHING
 Head action
 Arm action
 Hand action
KICKING
 Arm-trunk action
 Leg action

Check (✔) the appropriate box to show the developmental
level of body actions in the five selected
fundamental movement patterns.

I=Initial stage

E=Elementary stage

Class strengths:

M=Mature stage

Class weaknesses:

CLASS ABILITY CHART

NUMBER OF STUDENTS

0 1 2 3 4 5 6 7 8 9 10 11 12 13 14 15 16 17 18 19 20

INITIAL STAGE

Running   Leg action (side)
            Arm action
            Leg action (rear)

Jumping   Arm action
            Trunk action
            Leg-hip action

Throwing   Arm action
            Trunk action
            Leg-foot action

Catching   Head action
            Arm action
            Hand action

Kicking   Arm-trunk action
            Leg action

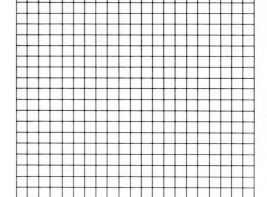

ELEMENTARY STAGE

Running   Leg action (side)
            Arm action
            Leg action (rear)

Jumping   Arm action
            Trunk action
            Leg-hip action

Throwing   Arm action
            Trunk action
            Leg-foot action

Catching   Head action
            Arm action
            Hand action

Kicking   Arm-trunk action
            Leg action

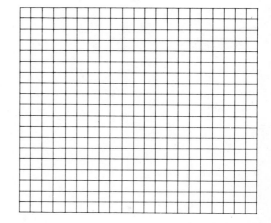

MATURE STAGE

Running   Leg action (side)
            Arm action
            Leg action (rear)

Jumping   Arm action
            Trunk action
            Leg-hip action

Throwing   Arm action
            Trunk action
            Leg-foot action

Catching   Head action
            Arm action
            Hand action

Kicking   Arm-trunk action
            Leg action

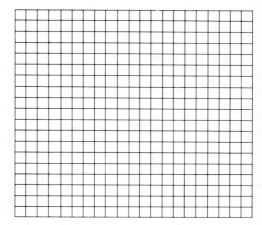

Graph the number of students in each class
who exhibit the various stages
(initial, elementary, and mature) for each
action of the five patterns.

NAME _____

INDIVIDUAL PROFILE

BIRTHDATE _____

	INITIAL STAGE	ELEMENTARY STAGE	MATURE STAGE

SUGGESTED MOVEMENT
EXPERIENCES

Running
    Leg action (side)
    Arm action
    Leg action (rear)

Jumping
    Arm action
    Trunk action
    Leg-hip action

Throwing
    Arm action
    Trunk action
    Leg-foot action

Catching
    Head action
    Arm action
    Hand action

Kicking
    Arm-trunk action
    Leg action

_____
_____
_____
_____
_____
_____
_____
_____
_____
_____
_____

Check (✔) the appropriate box to show the stage of
functioning for each action of the five
fundamental movement patterns.

Individual strengths:

Individual weaknesses:

INTERPRETING THE INFORMATION OBTAINED

Research indicates that school-age children should score at the mature level of functioning for all the movement patterns in this evaluation instrument. *With young children, however, individual differences in the rate of development must be considered.* It may be assumed that older children should have attained a mature level of functioning, and any deviation may be noted as a weakness in that particular pattern.

The information collected from this observational technique is subjective in nature; therefore, the results must be evaluated carefully. Results should show the relative strengths and weaknesses of a child's or group's fundamental movement patterns. Results may indicate certain activities for enhancing fundamental movement patterns and therefore may aid in curriculum planning or in individualizing instruction.

SUMMARY

The observational technique presented here has been designed to evaluate systematically the fundamental movement patterns of running, jumping, throwing, catching, and kicking. The developmental progressions of these patterns have been carefully constructed from current available literature and research on the development of movement during early childhood.

Sheets for evaluating movement patterns have been provided for each of the five patterns observed. The sample class and individual evaluation sheets are included to help the teacher summarize the information gathered with the use of this observational technique.

BIBLIOGRAPHY

The bibliographical references contained here represent supportive research information about the sequence of acquisition of five selected movement patterns. The bibliography has been divided into *Running, Jumping, Throwing, Catching,* and *Kicking.*

Running

1. Anderson, Norma M., and Randall, Florence C.: An Experimental Study of Factors Which Influence Speed in Running. Unpublished master's thesis, University of Wisconsin, 1931, p. 50.
2. Beck, Marjorie Catherine: The Path of the Center of Gravity During Running in Boys Grades One to Six. Unpublished doctoral dissertation, University of Wisconsin, 1965, pp. 115–20.
3. Clouse, Florence Cuthill: A Kinematic Analysis of the Development of the Running Patterns of Preschool Boys. Unpublished doctoral dissertation, University of Wisconsin, 1959, pp. 208–10.
4. Dittmer, Joann A.: A Kinematic Analysis of the Development of Running Patterns of Grade School Girls and Certain Factors Which Distinguish Good and Poor Performance at Observed Ages. Unpublished master's thesis, University of Wisconsin, 1962, pp. 18, 184–85.
5. Espenschade, Anna S., and Eckert, Helen M.: *Motor Development.* Columbus, Ohio: Charles E. Merrill, 1967, p. 110.

6. Felton, Elvira Amelia: A Kinesiological Comparison of Good and Poor Performers in the Standing Broad Jump. Unpublished master's thesis, University of Wisconsin, 1960, 73 pp.
7. Fortney, Virginia L.: The Swinging Limb in Running of Boys Ages Seven Through Eleven. Unpublished master's thesis, University of Wisconsin, 1964, 166 pp.
8. Gallahue, David, Werner, Peter, and Luedke, George: *A Conceptual Approach to Moving and Learning.* New York: John Wiley, 1975, p. 85.
9. Glassow, Ruth B., Halverson, Lolas E., and Rarick, G. Lawrence: *Improvement of Motor Development and Physical Fitness in Elementary School Children.* Cooperative Research Project No. 696, Cooperative Research Program of the Office of Education, U.S. Department of Health, Education, and Welfare and Wisconsin Alumni Research Foundation, p. 80.
10. Hardy, Richard E., and Gull, John B.: *Mental Retardation and Physical Disability.* Springfield, Ill.: Charles C Thomas, 1974, pp. 115–20.
11. Kay, Harry: The Development of Motor Skills from Birth to Adolescence. *Principles of Skill Acquisition,* Ed. E. A. Bilodeau. New York: Academic Press, 1969.
12. Rarick, G. Lawrence: *Motor Development During Infancy and Childhood.* Madison, Wis.: College Printing and Typing Co., 1961, p. 52.
13. Sinclair, Caroline B.: *Movement of the Young Child: Ages Two to Six.* Columbus, Ohio: Charles E. Merrill, 1973, pp. 29–32, 35.
14. Wickstrom, Ralph L.: *Fundamental Motor Patterns.* Philadelphia: Lea and Febiger, 1977, pp. 37–57.

Jumping

1. Cooper, John M., and Glassow, Ruth B.: *Kinesiology.* St. Louis: C. V. Mosby Co., 1972, pp. 220, 227, 229, 230.
2. Espenschade, Anna S., and Eckert, Helen M.: *Motor Development.* Columbus, Ohio: Charles E. Merrill, 1967, p. 115.
3. Felton, Elvira Amelia: A Kinesiological Comparison of Good and Poor Performers in the Standing Broad Jump. Unpublished master's thesis, University of Wisconsin, 1960, p. 60.
4. Glassow, Ruth B., Halverson, Lolas E., and Rarick, G. Lawrence: *Improvement of Motor Development and Physical Fitness in Elementary School Children.* Cooperative Research Project No. 696, Cooperative Research Program of the Office of Education, U.S. Department of Health, Education, and Welfare and Wisconsin Alumni Research Foundation, p. 80.
5. Guttridge, Mary V.: A study of motor achievements of young children. *Archives of Psychology, 244:*65, 165, 1939.
6. Halverson, Lolas E.: Development of motor patterns in young children. *Quest VI, A Symposium on Motor Learning, 6,* 4, 10, 1966.
7. Rarick, G. Lawrence: *Motor Development During Infancy and Childhood.* Madison, Wis.: College Printing and Typing Co., 1961, pp. 54, 55.
8. Wickstrom, Ralph L.: *Fundamental Motor Patterns.* Philadelphia: Lea and Febiger, 1977, pp. 59–90.
9. Wilson, Marjorie: *Development of Jumping Skill in Children.* Unpublished doctoral dissertation, State University of Iowa, 1945, pp. 48–50.
10. Zimmerman, Helen Margaret: Characteristic Likenesses and Differences Between Skilled and Non-skilled Performance of the Standing Long Jump. Unpublished doctoral dissertation, University of Wisconsin, 1951, pp. 141–42.

Throwing

1. Brophy, Kathleen J.: A Kinesiological Study of the Improvement in Motor Skill. Unpublished doctoral dissertation, University of Wisconsin, 1948, p. 158.
2. Corbin, Charles (ed.): *A Textbook of Motor Development.* Dubuque, Iowa: William C. Brown, 1973, p. 73.
3. Deach, Dorothy F.: Genetic Development of Motor Skills in Children Two Through Six Years of Age. Unpublished doctoral dissertation, University of Michigan, 1951, pp. 80–86, 90–91.
4. Guttridge, Mary V.: A study of motor achievements of young children. *Archives of Psychology, 244:*1–178, 1939.
5. Jones, Fredda Goodwin: A Descriptive and Mechanical Analysis of Throwing Skills of Children. Unpublished master's thesis, University of Wisconsin, 1951, pp. 85–86.

6. Keogh, Jack: Motor Performance of Elementary School Children. Los Angeles: University of California Department of Physical Education, 1965, p. 50.
7. Rarick, G. Lawrence: *Motor Development During Infancy and Childhood.* Madison, Wis.: College Printing and Typing Co., 1961, p. 57.
8. Wickstrom, Ralph L.: *Fundamental Motor Patterns.* Philadelphia: Lea and Febiger, 1977, pp. 91–117.
9. Wild, Monica: The behavior pattern of throwing and some observations concerning its course of development in children. *Research Quarterly, 9:22, 28, 33, 1938.*

Catching

1. Bruce, Russell D.: The Effects of Variations in Ball Trajectory upon the Catching Performance of Elementary School Children. Unpublished doctoral dissertation, University of Wisconsin, 1966, p. 128.
2. Cratty, Bryant J.: *Motor Ability and the Education of Retards.* Philadelphia: Lea and Febiger, 1969, p. 58.
3. Deach, Dorothy, F.: Genetic Development of Motor Skills in Children Two Through Six Years of Age. Unpublished doctoral dissertation, University of Michigan, 1951, pp. 93, 103–11.
4. Espenschade, Anna S., and Eckert, Helen M.: *Motor Development.* Columbus, Ohio: Charles E. Merrill, 1967, pp. 126–27.
5. Guttridge, Mary V.: A study of motor achievements of young children. *Archives of Psychology, 244:167, 1939.*
6. Victors, Evelyn Eloise: A Cinematographical Analysis of Catching Behavior of a Selected Group of Seven and Nine Year Old Boys. Unpublished doctoral dissertation, University of Wisconsin, 1961, p. 127.
7. Wellman, Beth L.: Motor achievement of pre-school children, *Childhood Education, 13:311–16, 1937.*
8. Wickstrom, Ralph L.: *Fundamental Motor Patterns.* Philadelphia: Lea and Febiger, 1977, pp. 119–142.

Kicking

1. Deach, Dorothy F.: Genetic Development of Motor Skills in Children Two Through Six Years of Age. Unpublished doctoral dissertation, University of Michigan, 1951, pp. 134–37, 142.
2. Halverson, Lolas E., and Roberton, M. A.: A Study of Motor Pattern Development in Young Children. National Convention of American Association of Health, Physical Education, and Recreation, 1966.
3. Wickstrom, Ralph L.: *Fundamental Motor Patterns.* Philadelphia: Lea and Febiger, 1977, pp. 177–206.

CHAPTER 7

ORGANIZING AND IMPLEMENTING THE MOTOR DEVELOPMENT PROGRAM

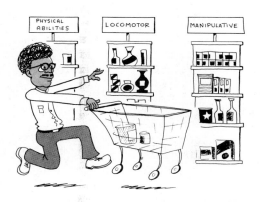

Many children experience difficulty in performing mature fundamental movement patterns. As noted previously, it is essential that these children be identified as soon as possible during the early childhood period. These children of low motor ability often can be helped to develop more efficient movements through an enrichment program of remedial activities.

Because the psychomotor needs of children vary greatly, the reader should use the material in this chapter only as a general guide for formulating a developmental or remedial program. Programs should be individually designed to satisfy the needs of the children to be served.

This chapter supplies the reader with the basic information necessary for providing young children with activities to improve their fundamental movement abilities. Material to be covered includes designing and implementing the program, structure of the remedial program, and sample movement experiences.

ORGANIZING THE PROGRAM

The motor development program should continually supply children with movement experiences to help them achieve their maximum level of functioning within their level of ability. This program should be provided for both young and older children who cannot benefit from other programs of physical activity and are often labeled "clumsy," "awkward," or "uncoordinated." Depending upon its design and intent, this program may involve one child or a group of children.

PROGRAM STRUCTURE

The person attempting to design a motor development program often faces numerous problems that include insufficient time to conduct the program, lack of equipment, limited facilities, and securing an effective, dependable staff. The success of the program depends, to a large degree, upon how these problems are approached and solved.

Because of insufficient time during school hours, the activities of the motor development program should usually be held immediately after school, approximately two days a week. Each lesson should last no longer than 1 hour to avoid boring and tiring the children.

If a large number of children are to be enrolled in the program, it will be necessary to group them according to their psychomotor needs, as well as their cognitive and affective levels. In order to provide individualized instruction, which is essential, there should be a small student-instructor ratio for each group of children. This often necessitates the use of volunteers for the program staff. It is vital to the continuity of the program that these individuals be reliable, knowledgeable about the development of children, and eager to work with and help children. Volunteers may often be recruited from organizations of parents, teachers, senior citizens, mature high school students, and college students majoring in physical education, early childhood education, and elementary education.

Because there is limited time for each lesson, each activity should be thoroughly planned and efficiently presented. Movement experiences should be structured so that each child participates fully. Activities that require children to stand in line or wait long periods of time to participate should be avoided. Through the use of inexpensive and homemade equipment, an attempt should be made to provide each child with his or her own piece of equipment. Parents can help collect items, such as plastic bottles, yarn, and rope, that can be used to construct equipment; they may also become interested in constructing large pieces of equipment.

Often programs are not initiated because of inadequate facilities. Within most communities there are many locations that have enough space for operation of a remedial program. Programs with small enrollments require little space to be conducted efficiently, but larger programs need additional space to accommodate the increased enrollment. Elementary schools often have multipurpose rooms that are not used after school hours. Churches, in many instances, have large rooms with adequate floor space, while most YMCA's, YWCA's, and Boy's Clubs have gymnasiums. Ideally, the motor development program should have both sufficient outdoor areas and an adequate indoor facility to accommodate the program's enrollment.

PROGRAM IMPLEMENTATION

Once the initial problems of design have been solved, the program must be implemented. The initial step in this process is making the community aware of the program and its objectives. This can often be accomplished by speaking to organizations concerned with children who have various impairments. During this initial stage of implementing the program, a mailing list should be compiled that includes possible children for the program, potential volunteers, teachers, school administrators, and local physicians. Local pediatricians in particular are invaluable for identifying children who have a motor impairment. In addition, local newspapers are usually willing to advertise a remedial program, and radio and television stations help reach parents through public service announcements.

Several months before the program starts, information and applications should be distributed to interested parents and individuals. Enrollment should be on a "first come, first serve" basis and should be restricted to a number that can be easily handled within the limitations of the program. During the first year of the program, enrollment should be especially limited so that unanticipated problems may be easily solved.

The program director should, if possible, charge a small fee for entrance into the program, unless it is supported financially through the school system or some other agency. This fee should not be intended to restrict enrollment but rather to serve two main purposes: (1) to cultivate and maintain parental interest (the parent who pays for instruction is more likely to be concerned that his or her child receives that instruction) and (2) to cover the expenses of the program.

All volunteers and instructors of the program should attend an organizational workshop several weeks before the first program session. Policies and procedures of the program should be discussed as well as each person's role in the program.

Once enrolled, each child should be scheduled for assessment prior to the first week of the program. This evaluation should determine how well the child performs fundamental movements and physical skills. Information on matters such as self concept may provide instructors with additional information about the child's needs. Parents should be informed of the results of this evaluation and given recommendations regarding their role in improving their child's motor ability.

An attempt should be made to group children according to their needs and developmental levels. Each group should be limited to five to eight children, with several instructors assigned to each group. Color-coded name tags have proved helpful in organizing children into these groups.

LESSON DESIGN

Enrollment determines the manner in which the motor development program is structured. Programs with a limited number of children can be more informally structured than those with many students. Large programs require a great deal of cooperation between instructors. The person designing and implementing the program must determine its organizational framework.

PLANNING ACTIVITIES

It is essential that each lesson be thoroughly planned and that the instructors adapt the proposed activities to fulfill the needs of the children in their particular group. Complete activity plans should be available for each instructor at least one week before that lesson is to be taught. This lesson outline should include the specific objectives of each movement experience, a brief description of the activity, suggested adaptations, and special points to emphasize for each activity.

Table 7-1 SAMPLE LESSON ACTIVITY AREAS

ACTIVITY STATION NUMBER	AREA OF CONCENTRATION	ACTIVITIES DESIGNED TO ENHANCE
1	Locomotor movements	Running, jumping, leaping, galloping, hopping, skipping
2	Physical abilities	Strength, agility, flexibility, stability
3	Manipulative movements	Throwing, catching, kicking, striking, bouncing, rolling
4	Open	Perceptual-motor skills, fine motor skills, "quiet time" activities, rhythms

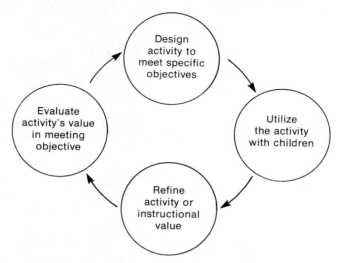

Figure 7–1   Steps in developing appropriate movement experiences.

Portions of each lesson should be devoted to enhancing specific components of fundamental movement. Programs composed of several groups of children may operate well by using the principle of circuit training. Groups may be rotated through a sequence of activity stations, each emphasizing a particular area of fundamental movement. Table 7–1 shows how activity stations may be organized.

When deciding upon movement experiences for each activity station, a person should (1) develop an activity to achieve a specific objective, (2) use the activity with the children, (3) evaluate how well the activity satisfies the desired objective, and (4) revise the activity or instructional strategy, or both, accordingly (Figure 7–1). Although the initial development of activities takes a great deal of time and effort, the program, once established, may be used for years and improved with continuous reevaluation and addition of new material.

INSTRUCTIONAL AIDS

The instructional strategies used in the remedial motor development program may differ somewhat from those of the developmental program. Older children lagging behind in motor development often need a more focused teaching approach than younger children developing normally. The instructor must always attempt to promote the best learning behavior of the children by using the most effective and efficient teaching methods. Various audio-visual aids, for example, have proved useful in enhancing fundamental movement of young children. These materials can often be used to help individualize instruction.

The use of video tape provides the instructor with a valuable means of

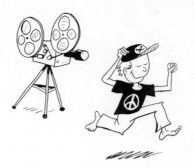

analyzing children's motor performance. Children can be taped while executing a movement, and the quality of the performance can be thoroughly evaluated. Video tape can also give the performer immediate visual feedback on the quality of movement. Children can thus analyze their own performance and become aware of common faults in their movement.

Advances in movie film during the past several years have made the use of this visual aid feasible. Many Super 8 movie cameras, for instance, can shoot film at faster than normal speeds and, therefore, slow the projected image. Slow motion film can demonstrate mature movements to children who are having difficulty in correcting common faults in their patterns.

A person familiar with the basics of motion picture photography can easily develop a series of demonstration films for instructional purposes. There are a wide variety of films currently available, and new automatic cameras enable even the novice to produce films of good quality. Film may be processed, edited, and used with a regular Super 8 projector, or it may be put into cartridge form to be shown in Super 8 loop film projectors.*

The instructor can also use auditory prompting to help children perform mature movement patterns. These cues can be classified as either *quality words* or *action words*. Quality words describe and emphasize correct form, whereas action words may enable children to better understand a movement. Table 7–2 is a sample list of action and quality words.

Various pieces of equipment can help children to correctly position their bodies in preparation for performing a movement. Paper footprints, hoops, lines, ropes, and cones can all be used to structure movement activities. Figure 7–2 shows examples of how cut-out footprints can visually represent some specific fundamental movements.

Posters that demonstrate the mature patterns of movement reinforce verbal directions. On the poster each movement may be divided into three

---

*Further information can be obtained from Technicolor, Customer Service Dept., P.O. Box 4, Springfield, Massachusetts 01101.

Table 7–2 EXAMPLES OF AUDITORY CUES

QUALITY WORDS	*ACTION WORDS*
Swing = steady	Flex at the hips
Hard = soft	Completely extend the legs
Hold = release	Step with the foot
Fast = slow	Swing from the hips
Backward = forward	Control with the fingers
Large = small	

phases—preparatory, action, and follow-through—and specific points should be emphasized in each phase. Figure 7–3 is a poster designed to assist children experiencing difficulty with the standing long jump pattern.

SUMMARY

The manner in which the program is organized and implemented determines its success to a large degree. The motor development program should continually provide children with enriching movement experiences. Planning such a program involves establishing its general objectives and developing its policies and procedures.

Activities should be designed to achieve a specific objective; after being utilized, they should then be evaluated and restructured to more fully satisfy that objective. To increase the effectiveness of the movement experiences, instructors are encouraged to experiment with various types of audio-visual aids. It must be emphasized that not all activities or instructional strategies are successful with all children. Therefore, the instructor must constantly modify activities to fulfill the psychomotor needs of the children.

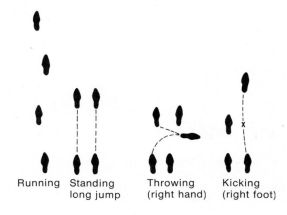

Figure 7–2 Cut-out footprints representing various fundamental movements.

Running   Standing long jump   Throwing (right hand)   Kicking (right foot)

Standing Long Jump

Start   Takeoff

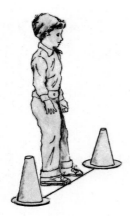 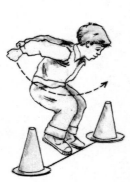 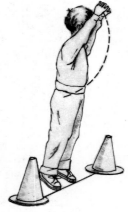

Begin by standing behind the cones, toes on the line and feet approximately a shoulder width apart.

Swing your arms backward as you bend at the waist, keeping your head up. The knees should then be bent until you feel comfortable (never more than 90°).

Swing your arms forward as hard as you can and extend your legs completely. Lean as far forward as you can.

Flight   Landing

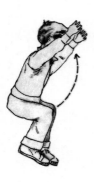 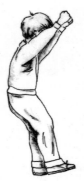 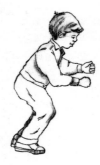

Keep your arms high and attempt to pull your knees to your chest.

Before making contact with the ground, extend your legs. Hit the ground with your heels first.

Absorb the shock of landing with your legs and reach forward with your arms.

Figure 7–3   Example of a poster illustrating the standing long jump pattern.

BIBLIOGRAPHY

1. Kemp, Jerrold E.: *Planning and Producing Audiovisual Materials.* New York: Thomas Y. Crowell, 1975, 320 pp.
2. Minor, Ed, and Frye, Harvey R.: *Techniques for Producing Visual Instructional Media.* New York: McGraw-Hill, 1970, 305 pp.

CHAPTER 8

METHODS OF TEACHING FUNDAMENTAL MOVEMENT

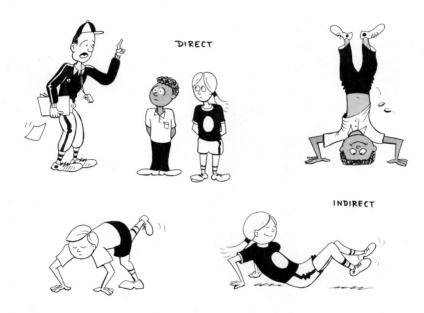

The sequential development of mature patterns of movement involves complex interaction between maturation and experience. In creating movement activities for children, we must recognize this fact, which we have dealt with in detail in discussing the acquisition and assessment of fundamental movement patterns. We must also be concerned with *how* we can effectively interact with children by using a variety of teaching approaches before we can determine *what* types of movement experiences are best suited to children at various stages of development.

In recent years there has been a proliferation of materials dealing with styles of teaching. Probably the best known work is *Teaching: From Command to Discovery*[7] by Muska Mosston. His excellent text describes a spectrum of teaching styles ranging from the most direct, or command, method to the most indirect, or exploratory, method. It is not our intent to dwell on methodology for teaching motor skills, but a brief description and discussion of indirect and direct methods of teaching motor skills is presented in this chapter. Practical suggestions for using problem-solving techniques to develop mature patterns of movement are also included.

TEACHING APPROACHES

Teaching is a learned behavior, and as such it is susceptible to modification. The manner in which we interact with children to help them learn is influenced by many conditions. Considerations about teachers, children, and environment help determine which teaching method or methods should be included in the lesson. Such things as the teacher's personality, expertise, values, and learning goals influence the choice of methodology. The child's maturity, learning behavior, and interest also must be taken into account as well as environmental factors such as available facilities, equipment, time, and safety. Table 8–1 lists several of these determining factors.

Basically, teaching methodologies range from those that are direct, or teacher-centered, to those that are indirect, or child-centered. Figure 8–1 illustrates the relationship between direct and indirect approaches. It is our

Table 8–1 FACTORS AFFECTING THE SELECTION OF VARIOUS TEACHING METHODS

TEACHER FACTORS	CHILD FACTORS	ENVIRONMENTAL FACTORS
Personality	Age	Facilities
Ability	Maturity	Equipment
Philosophy	Readiness	Materials
Values	Learning style	Time allotted
Objectives	Interest	Weather
Interest	Ability	Type of activity
		Safety

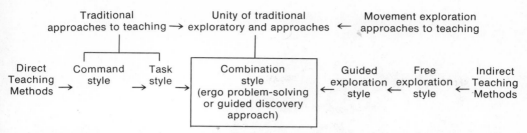

Figure 8–1 The scope of teaching styles and the link between direct and indirect teaching methods.

opinion that very few, if any, teachers of children use any one particular teaching style to the exclusion of all others. Instead, the tendency is to use a variety of direct methods or indirect methods based on the factors outlined earlier. Teachers who favor direct approaches in teaching movement tend to use the command and task styles. Those who prefer more indirect approaches generally recommend free and guided exploration and problem-solving styles.

DIRECT TEACHING METHODS

Direct methods of teaching movement skills are the traditional teaching approaches that have been used by physical educators and classroom teachers for hundreds of years. These methods are teacher-centered because the teacher makes all or most of the decisions concerning what, how, and when the student is to perform. Direct methods have many advantages. They are efficient and focused and leave little opportunity for error. The structured learning environment is conducive to good class control. Direct methods are also easy to use with individuals or with large groups of children. However, the disadvantages of direct teaching methods are many. They do not allow for much individuality and inventiveness on the part of the learner. They are more concerned with the goal or product of the learning experience than the process of learning involved. Direct methods also make little allowance for individual differences. They are based on the false assumption that all children have reached about the same level of learning and progress at the same rate.

Although direct methods of teaching often have disadvantages, especially with young children, they may be necessary (Fig. 8–2) and can be modified in a variety of ways. Both verbal and nonverbal communication techniques may be altered significantly by the teacher. The manner in which the class is conducted need not take on a "drill-sergeant" atmosphere but may rather be one in which duties, responsibilities, and privileges are shared, with the teacher still making the key decisions. The command and the task approaches are the two most popular types of direct teaching methods.

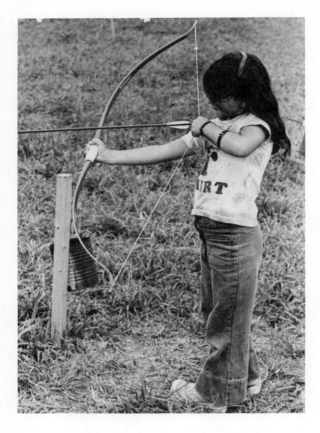

Figure 8–2 In some instances it is necessary to utilize a direct teaching approach.

THE COMMAND APPROACH

The command approach to teaching movement skills is the classic method of teaching movement skills. It consists of (1) a short explanation and demonstration of the skill to be performed, (2) student practice prior to giving further directions or pointing out specific errors, (3) general comments to the class about their performance, (4) further explanation and demonstration, if necessary, (5) student practice with "coaching hints" to individuals or groups having difficulty, and (6) implementation of the skill in a game or a rhythmical or self-testing activity.

The command approach makes all of the pre-performance and performance decisions for the learner. The teacher rigidly controls what is to be practiced, how it is to be done, and when to start and stop.

THE TASK APPROACH

The task approach to teaching movement is similar to the command approach because the teacher still controls what is to be practiced and how it is to be performed. However, in using the task approach, the teacher does permit a degree of decision-making on the part of the child. A greater amount of freedom and flexibility is introduced into the learning environment. The children are given more responsibility for themselves but are not permitted to choose what to do or how to do their assigned task.

When using the task approach, the teacher follows a sequence of (1) explanation and demonstration of different levels of the task to be performed by the class or individuals (task cards of varying difficulty in written or pictorial form may also be distributed), (2) practice of the designated task by students at their own pace and at their particular level of ability, (3) help for individuals or groups having difficulty and challenges to advanced students to achieve higher levels of performance.

The task style permits the child to work at his group level of ability. It may be undertaken on an individual, reciprocal, or small basis. An individual may work alone at the task provided by the teacher and evaluate himself, or he may work with a partner who assesses his performance. Students may also work together in groups of three or four on a specific task, with one performing, a second evaluating, and a third recording the students' performance of the task. The task method is a direct teaching approach, but less so than the command method.

INDIRECT TEACHING METHODS

Indirect methods of teaching movement skills came into vogue in North America during the early 1960's. Various indirect teaching approaches had been advocated prior to that time, but it was not until the works of Rudolph Laban[6] and Liselott Diem[3] found their way to North America that educators began to look seriously at the potential for using indirect teaching approaches in motor skill development.

These indirect approaches were initially rejected by many physical educators steeped in the direct methods of command and task teaching. Soon, however, there was a distinct division between those who have come to be known as "traditional physical educators" and those called "movement educators." Each group claimed that their methods of teaching movement skills were best.

There has recently been a mellowing of points of view, and many educators, rather than identifying with *either* direct or indirect methods, are recognizing the tremendous value of both types of teaching approaches. There has been a shift of focus from the method to the learner. In trying to gear their methods of instruction to the child rather than making the child suit the methods, educators are increasingly eclectic in their choice of teaching approaches. As a result, indirect teaching approaches have finally won their place in the spectrum of teaching approaches used in physical education. They do not automatically insure optimal learning any more than direct approaches do. They do, however, provide the learner with greater opportunity for freedom and assumption of responsibility within the educational setting (Fig. 8–3).

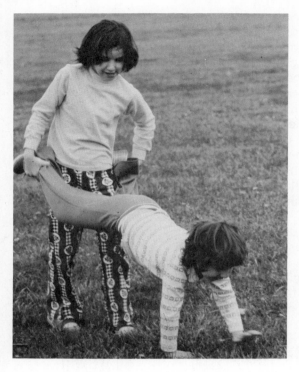

Figure 8–3 Indirect methods allow the student considerable freedom in setting goals.

Among the advantages of indirect methods is that they permit the student considerable freedom in setting goals and determining how these goals are going to be accomplished. In other words, the learner becomes more involved in the learning process by being given opportunity and encouragement to explore and experiment in a variety of ways. Another important advantage of indirect teaching approaches is that they allow for individual differences between learners. Each student is able to find a degree of success in a movement performance at his or her particular level of ability.

The disadvantages of indirect teaching methods are mainly that they are time-consuming and that teachers unfamiliar with the techniques often find them difficult to use productively. Indirect approaches require considerable patience on the part of the teacher. Plenty of time must be permitted for experimentation, trial and error, and question asking. Because some teachers have not been trained in the techniques involved, they find indirect methods difficult to use. They often have trouble maintaining class control, structuring challenging situations or problems, and providing for continuity both within lessons and between lessons. These disadvantages do not mean, however, that indirect methods are inferior to direct methods of teaching movement. On the contrary, indirect methods do play a very important role in motor development, particularly at the preschool and primary grade level. The two major indirect methods of teaching used today are the movement exploration approach and the problem-solving or combination approach.

MOVEMENT EXPLORATION

The exploratory approach to teaching movement requires the teacher to design broad-based movement tasks having no one particular solution. Any *reasonable* solution of the task by the student is considered acceptable. The teacher neither demonstrates how to perform the action, nor presents a detailed verbal description of it. The student is given the opportunity to perform the movement as he sees fit. By focusing primarily on the learning process itself rather than the product of learning, the exploratory approach does not emphasize form or precision; nor does it require that each child performs the activity in the same manner. The teacher is interested, however, in providing meaningful movement tasks in which each child is encouraged to explore the movement potential of his body, develop fundamental movement abilities, find success at his level of ability, and express himself in a creative manner.

Movement exploration may be totally free or guided by the teacher. The use of **free exploration** permits the child to move in any way he wishes, as long as it is safe. Free exploration is the most indirect form of teaching. Two sample commands are: "Do anything you wish with this ball" and "move any way you want to on the balance beam." This extreme form of indirect teaching has been used to the exclusion of other forms by some in the name of progressive education and has thus caused many to reject it as a viable method of teaching. Free exploration can be valuable in the *initial stages* of learning, but it is considerably limited in its breadth and scope and should be followed by guided exploration.

Guided exploration permits the learner plenty of expression, creativity, and experimentation but somewhat restricts how the learner may respond to the movement tasks presented. A wide variety of responses are still encouraged, but the presentation of the task is modified. For example, the teacher may now say, "See how many ways you can *bounce* the ball," or "Move from one end of the balance beam to the other, often changing your direction (or level, speed, base of support, and so forth)." The child may explore many ways of accomplishing the tasks put to him.

THE COMBINATION APPROACH

The combination method uses both direct and indirect methods of teaching and attempts to include the best aspects of both. Children are permitted free and guided exploration, but may also be given specific skill instruction by way of the task or command approaches. The combination approach may be effectively used with both young and older children. We advocate using this approach with children in the development and refinement of their fundamental movement patterns because it recognizes both the individuality of each learner and the necessity for developing mature patterns of movement during the critical years of early and middle childhood.

Briefly, the combination approach involves a sequence of (1) free exploration, (2) guided exploration, (3) progressive problem-solving, and (4) specific skill instruction. The teacher first poses a general task to the student (free exploration). For example, the instructor may say, "Get the beanbag from one end of the room to the other any way you wish." Next, a few general restrictions are added, and the command may be modified to: "See how many ways you can get the beanbag across the room while remaining in one spot." Guided exploration remarks such as this are then followed by a series of questions, challenges, or problems posed to the student (problem-solving). Each problem is stated in such a way that the learner's response possibilities lead directly to the desired skill. For example, "Using a throwing motion, see if you can get the beanbag across the room," may be followed by "Can you throw the beanbag overhand (underhand, and so on)?" and concluded with "How do we stand when we throw?" or "How do we make our bodies move when we want to throw as far as we can?" The teacher continually structures and restructures a variety of problems progressively more narrow in scope for the child to solve. Up to this point there is no explanation or demonstration of how to perform the overhand throwing pattern. After following the sequence of free exploration, guided exploration, and problem-solving, the teacher now incorporates specific skill instruction into the lesson for those who need it. Many perform the mature movement skill at this point. They may be grouped with those who are experiencing difficulty and instructed to work on the overhand throw using a small group or reciprocal method. Those having trouble may observe other students or the teacher perform the desired skill and they work on it under more direct supervision by the teacher.

The combination approach possesses the advantages of both the direct and indirect approaches and few of their disadvantages. The major disadvantages remaining are that it is time-consuming and takes practice on the part of the teacher to be perfect. These are outweighed, however, by the fact that each child is involved in the process of learning, exploring, experimenting, and finding success while still working toward the goal of higher skill levels. Figure 8–4 is a diagram of the combination approach to teaching fundamental movement skills.

As explained earlier, the combination approach is more heavily weighted toward specific skill instruction when the teacher is working on remedial movement pattern development with older or atypical children. With preschool and primary grade children, the problem-solving component of the combination approach is generally more stressed.

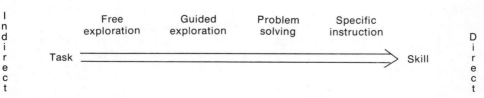

Figure 8–4   Anatomy of the combination approach to teaching movement skills.

PROBLEM-SOLVING AND MOVEMENT PATTERN DEVELOPMENT

It is easy to read about a variety of teaching styles and to gain a textbook knowledge of how and when each method can be appropriately applied. This textbook knowledge, however, is no substitute for experience. It is relatively easy to master the command and task forms of teaching described in the previous section; most of us have been exposed to these methods throughout our education career. Incorporating movement exploration, especially in its free form, into actual lessons is also fairly simple because teacher involvement is minimal. The use of problem-solving, however, is quite another matter. Most of us are not as well acquainted with this technique and have had little opportunity to observe others using it. Therefore, it is the purpose of this section to offer practical suggestions in planning and implementing the movement lesson by utilizing a combination approach that emphasizes problem-solving. Chapter 9 presents a variety of movement activities suitable for use with this technique. The reader is cautioned, however, to recognize that no amount of textbook learning develops a good teacher. Only frequent and regular practice with children is of any real and lasting benefit.

PLANNING THE LESSON

Careful planning of lessons is of crucial importance. Chapter 5 deals with considerations about curriculum, and the reader is referred to it for careful review. Before actually planning the lesson the teacher must make several determinations about the level of psychomotor development and the cognitive and affective maturity of the learner. Given this information and knowledge of available facilities, equipment, time allotted, and other important information, the teacher is free to determine the specific objectives of the movement lesson.

The primary objectives of the lesson concerned with fundamental movement patterns are the development and refinement of specific movement abilities and physical abilities. These objectives may be stated simply in terms of the learner's expected goal. Care should be taken to make sure that this goal is suitable for the child's stage of pattern development, be it initial, elementary, or mature. For example, in planning the lesson the objective may be "to improve jumping ability in the jump for distance" or "to be able to catch a small ball with greater efficiency."

Once the learning goal has been established, the teacher proceeds to formulate the initial task and subsequent problems to be presented in the lesson itself. Initially the tasks should be open-ended and exploratory. They should allow for a limited amount of free exploration followed by guided exploration and problem-solving. The problem-solving portion of the lesson should directly lead to refinement of the desired pattern by insuring that each succeeding problem or question given to the learner is more narrowly defined. The teacher should attempt to anticipate the broad range of possible responses before presenting the problems in the lesson itself. It takes practice to structure meaningful challenges that lead to progressive skill refinement. The teacher should be prepared for solutions other than those anticipated and should recognize the necessity for restructuring problems that are not clearly understood initially.

In planning the lesson, the teacher needs to consider also at what point to intervene with more direct forms of teaching. Following the problem-solving portion of the lesson, the instructor must decide whether to use small group, reciprocal, or individual task instruction or command instruction.

The teacher must next determine which specific games, rhythms, or self-testing activities that make use of the movement pattern are to be incorporated into the lesson. The teacher may decide, for example, to have the children play a circle or tag game to reinforce the running pattern worked on in the lesson; or he may select a rhythmical activity with a fast tempo to permit rhythmical running.

The last part of lesson planning concerns the summary and review. It is important for the teacher to sit down with the children at the end of the lesson and review the movement skills worked on. This summary reinforces the movement concepts dealt with and crystalizes them in the children's thinking and action.

The steps to be followed in planning the motor development lesson are briefly outlined below:

1. Determine the level of motor development.
2. Determine cognitive and affective maturity.
3. Inventory available facilities, equipment, and space.
4. State the specific objectives of the lesson.
5. Decide on the initial task to be presented to the class (free exploration).
6. Determine subsequent open-ended tasks to be presented to the class (guided exploration).
7. Develop a list of movement problems progressing from very general challenges to more narrowly defined ones (problem-solving).
8. Decide at what point to incorporate more direct methods and determine the approach to be used (small group, reciprocal, or individual task or command instruction).
9. Incorporate appropriate games, rhythms, or self-testing activities into the lesson.
10. Decide what will be summarized and reviewed at the end of the lesson and how it will be done.

IMPLEMENTING THE LESSON

When implementing the fundamental movement lesson, the teacher needs to be aware of several factors. First, it is important to have an understanding of the basic body mechanics of each skill. In order to foster efficient development of fundamental movement abilities, the instructor must understand the principles of movement involved and how to apply them.

Second, the teacher must be sure that children are in fact making progress toward accomplishing the specific objectives of the lesson. It is not enough that each child is simply active. It must be activity designed for the purpose of achieving the lesson objectives. The teacher, therefore, will find it necessary to continually structure new problems and restructure old ones at a pace suitable for both the rapid learner and the slower learner.

A third factor to consider is safety. The teacher must be constantly concerned with whether safety precautions in the lesson are being followed or ignored. Return to a more direct approach may be temporarily necessary during the problem-solving portion of the lesson in order to remedy an unsafe situation quickly and efficiently.

Fourth, the teacher should circulate throughout the class during the lesson and structure problems in a variety of ways. Problems may take the form of questions, challenges, discussions, or verbal cues and should be varied so that none is used to the exclusion of the others. Phrases such as Who can? How can you?, Find a way, Let's see if, and Is there another way to? are helpful in constructing the problem. Care must be taken not to ververbalize at the expense of active involvement on the part of the children.

A fifth and final factor to consider in implementing the lesson is activity itself. Children have a great need to be active. Thus the motor development lesson should be one of *active learning,* not learning with little or no activity.

Success in using the combination approach to teaching movement depends on careful adherence to the planning and implementation factors discussed previously as well as the teacher's genuine interest, enthusiasm, experience, ingenuity, and imaginative approach to teaching movement. To summarize, five crucial factors in implementing the movement lesson are:

1. Knowing basic principles of movement.
2. Insuring that steady progress is being made.
3. Enforcing safety regulations.
4. Circulating throughout the class and using a variety of verbal formats to present the problems.
5. Providing vigorous activity continuously.

SUMMARY

A variety of teaching approaches are required for successful incorporation of movement experiences into the child's day. A number of factors regarding teachers, children and environment need to be considered prior to selecting appropriate teaching styles.

Teaching methods may be divided into two broad categories, direct and indirect. The command and task approaches to teaching movement represent the direct or traditional methods of teaching. Both are very popular and have been widely used for many years.

The movement exploration approach, using both free and guided exploration, is an indirect method of teaching movement that has become popular in recent years. The combination approach, also an indirect method, represents a compromise between the extremes of indirect and direct teaching. It utilizes a problem-solving approach in conjunction with other techniques and is advocated as an ideal method for developing fundamental movement abilities. Careful consideration of a number of planning and implementation factors and practice in the use of the combination method leads to successful lessons.

BIBLIOGRAPHY

1. Barrett, Kate: *Exploration: A Method of Teaching Movement.* Madison, Wis.: College Printing and Typing Co., 1965.
2. Cope, John: *Discovery Methods in Physical Education.* London: Nelson and Sons, 1967.
3. Diem, Liselott: *Who Can?* Frankfurt: William Lippert, 1955.
4. Gilliom, Bonnie: *Basic Movement Education: Rationale and Teaching Units.* Reading, Mass.: Addison-Wesley, 1971.
5. Heitman, Helen, and Kneer, Marian E.: *Physical Education Instructional Techniques: An Individualized Humanistic Approach.* Englewood Cliffs, N.J.: Prentice-Hall, 1976.
6. Laban, Rudolph: *The Mastery of Movement.* London: MacDonald and Evans, 1960.
7. Mosston, Muska: *Teaching: From Command to Discovery.* Belmont, Calif.: Wadsworth, 1972.
8. Mosston, Muska: *Teaching Physical Education.* Columbus, Ohio: Charles E. Merrill, 1966.
9. Ryser, Otto: *A Teacher's Manual for Tumbling and Apparatus Stunts.* 5th ed. Dubuque, Iowa: William C. Brown, 1976.
10. Schurr, Evelyn: *Movement Experiences for Children.* Englewood Cliffs, N.J.: Prentice-Hall, 1975.

MOVEMENT EXPERIENCES

SECTION CONCEPTS

1. One's physical abilities and movement abilities interact to influence performance.
2. Indirect methods of teaching can be used to enhance physical abilities and movement abilities in young children.
3. Direct teaching methods may be used to enhance the basic movement patterns of older children.

CHAPTER 9

MOVEMENT EXPERIENCES FOR ENHANCING PHYSICAL ABILITIES

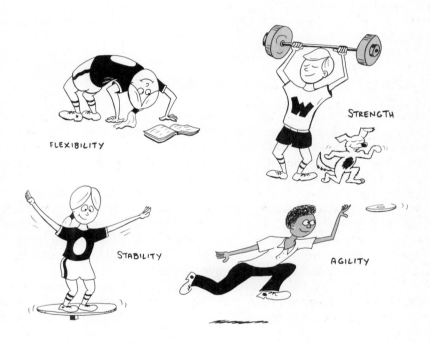

FLEXIBILITY

STRENGTH

STABILITY

AGILITY

The preceding three chapters dealt with designing and implementing a program to improve the fundamental movement patterns of young children. Before attempting to establish a series of developmental movement experiences for children, the reader should have a thorough understanding of these chapters.

This chapter presents a variety of movement activities for enhancing children's physical abilities, which include stability, agility, flexibility, and strength. The following chapters offer both developmental and remedial movement experiences for the basic patterns assessed by the observational tool in Chapter 6. Additional developmental activities for children who have already refined their fundamental movement abilities are also presented.

These chapters by no means list all the experiences that can be structured, but rather serve as examples of what can be developed. Individuals concerned with improving fundamental movement must supplement these activities with additional experiences and patterns when needed.

THE THREE DIMENSIONS OF MOVEMENT

Total motor development is an integration of three dimensions of movement. The first dimension, which is the primary concern of this text, is *fundamental movement abilities* (running, jumping, throwing, catching, and so forth). The first leg of the motor ability triangle (Fig. 9–1) represents fundamental movement abilities.

The second dimension of movement, represented by the second leg of the triangle, is *physical abilities.* Physical abilities are various qualities of physical and motor fitness, such as strength, agility, stability, flexibility, coordination, power, and so on. The development of these physical abilities should coincide with the development of the child's movement abilities so that the third dimension of movement can be attained.

This third dimension of movement represented as the apex of motor development, is *performance abilities.* One's performance abilities, whether they be qualitative (initial, elementary, mature) or quantitative

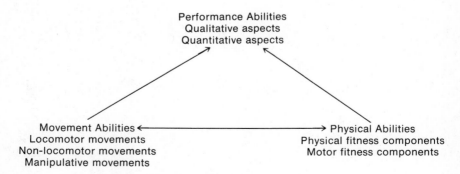

Figure 9–1   Motor ability triangle.

(distance covered, time elapsed), are affected by the interaction of one's movement abilities with one's physical abilities. With this important concept in mind, the teacher of fundamental movement should be concerned with developing the child's physical abilities in order to maximize his performance potential. Development of the child's fitness abilities should not be neglected. If the improvement of fitness is not emphasized, it is likely that there will be adverse effects on the level of the child's performance, in terms of both quality and quantity.

We must view this triangular concept of human movement from the standpoint of implementation. It is easy to draw a series of lines, use jargon, discuss the interrelated nature of movement, and construct a conceptual model. None of this is important, however, if both the teachers and the children are unable to translate the model into a workable form. It is the job of the teacher to make a conscious distinction between those movement experiences that enhance movement abilities and those that improve the child's physical ability. Would a child say, "Now I am building strength," or "Tomorrow I will work on my agility, and the following day I will practice running"? Probably not!

The teacher must determine how much of the lesson should be devoted to developing the child's movement abilities and how much to his physical abilities. The teacher must also be concerned with progression from simple to more complex activities and with the role of the lesson in the overall growth and development of the children being taught. The teacher should quickly recognize that many experiences incorporated into the movement lesson improve both movement and physical abilities and that a sound, developmentally based program makes positive contributions to children's performance of abilities.

ACTIVITIES FOR ENHANCING PHYSICAL ABILITIES

The following section deals with movement experiences designed specifically to promote the development of children's physical abilities. Balance, agility, flexibility, and strength are included because of their particularly close relationship to the fundamental movements dealt with in this text.

STABILITY

Stability is the most basic component of movement. It is a prerequisite to all efficient movement and must be regarded as an essential part of all fundamental movement abilities. Therefore, this physical ability must be developed to its maximum potential in each child.

Stability involves gaining and maintaining equilibrium in relation to the force of gravity when the body is placed in various positions. It also involves the ability to compensate rapidly and accurately for changes in balance with appropriate, measured body movement. The concept of stability encompasses the notions of static and dynamic balance and extends beyond to include any movement in which gaining and maintaining the equilibrium is a primary concern.

The following list is a collection of movement experiences for developing and refining the stability abilities of young children. The activities use only three types of equipment: balance beam, balance board, and inner tubes. Each type is easy to make or readily available. A variety of other equipment, such as coffee can stilts, balance blocks, ladders, benches, beanbags, and trampolines, may be used. The reader is referred to *Motor Development and Movement Experiences for Young Children (3–7)*[1] for a more comprehensive compilation of stability activities.

Challenge Activities on the Balance Beam

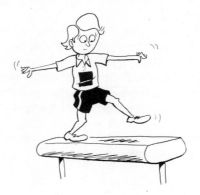

Can you. . .

1. walk forward on the beam with a follow step?
2. walk forward on the beam with a cross step?
3. walk sideways on the beam with a follow step?
4. walk sideways on the beam with a cross-over step?
5. walk to the center using one of the above steps and continue to the end using another?
6. walk to the end of the beam using one of the above steps, turn around, and return?
7. walk backward on the beam using a follow step?
8. walk backward on the beam using a cross step?
9. alternate forward, sideward, and backward walking with turning around on the beam?
10. walk fast from one end to the other using various steps?
11. walk slowly from one end to the other using various steps?
12. walk from one end of the beam to the other with the arms in various positions (up, out, down, and so on)?
13. walk from one end of the beam to the other using different body

positions (half squat, full squat, bending forward, bending backward, and so on)?
14. walk on your toes?
15. walk on your heels?
16. walk and make dip steps?
17. walk and pick up three (five, seven, and so forth) objects and carry
them to the end of the beam?
18. walk while holding a heavy object, such as a suitcase or pail of
water, in one hand?
19. walk and step over several objects?
20. walk and step under several objects?
21. walk and step through a hoop?
22. walk and combine going over, under, and through objects?
23. walk while carrying a long pole? A short pole? How do they differ
in helping you balance?
24. find different ways to get from one end of the beam to the other?
25. move with a partner on the beam?
26. walk on two beams and repeat many of the above activities?
27. can you catch a ball (beanbag, and so on) on the beam?
28. can you bounce and catch a ball while walking on the beam?
29. walk on all fours?
30. walk with your eyes closed?

Challenge Activities on the Balance Board

Can you. . .

1. balance on the board any way you can?
2. balance with your feet apart?
3. balance with your feet together?
4. balance with your legs straight?
5. balance with your legs bent?
6. balance in a squatted position?
7. balance with your hand touching the board?
8. balance with your head touching the board?
9. balance on one foot?
10. balance on your seat?
11. balance on three body parts?
12. balance with your arm in different positions (up, out, and down)?
13. find the best way to balance?
14. find the easiest way to balance?
15. find the hardest way to balance?
16. balance and look at me?
17. balance and look at John and then Susie?
18. balance and look across the room?
19. balance and look at the board?
20. balance with one eye closed?
21. balance with both eyes closed?

22. balance and toss and catch an object?
23. balance and catch an object from a partner?
24. balance and toss an object to a partner?
25. balance while bouncing and catching a ball?
26. balance while dribbling a ball?
27. step from one balance board to another?
28. balance with a partner on your balance board?
29. balance with a partner as long as you can?
30. balance with a partner and change positions while balancing?

Challenge Activities with Truck Inner Tubes

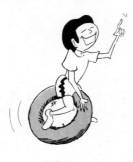

Can you. . .

1. stand on the inner tube?
2. walk on the inner tube?
3. walk in different directions?
4. crawl on the tube without falling off?
5. bounce on the tube with both feet?
6. bounce with your feet apart?
7. bounce with your feet together?
8. bounce and make a quarter turn?
9. bounce and turn halfway around?
10. bounce and move forward around the tube?
11. bounce and move sideways around the tube?
12. bounce and move backward around the tube?
13. bounce from one side of the tube to the center and then to the other side?
14. bounce on, off, and back on the tube in different ways?
15. step from one side of the tube to the other?
16. jump from one side of the tube to the other?
17. bounce from one side of the tube to the other?
18. bounce and look at me?
19. bounce while looking across the room?
20. bounce while looking from point to point?
21. bounce while looking at your feet?
22. bounce with your eyes closed?
23. bounce and catch a ball?
24. bounce and toss a ball?

25. bounce and toss a ball at a target or to a person?
26. bounce while bouncing and catching a ball?
27. bounce and toss and catch a ball?
28. bounce and dribble a ball?
29. bounce with a partner, repeating several of the activities just listed?
30. bounce in rhythmical opposition to your partner while holding hands with him?

AGILITY

Agility involves moving the body through space by an efficient combination of coordination and strength. Participation in movement activities requiring changes in body direction promotes the development of agility. The developmental program for young children should contain a variety of problem-solving activities of progressive difficulty that may be divided into three categories: those involving changes in body height, those involving changes in the distance through which the body is projected into space, and those involving changes in the direction of body movement. The movement activity ideas that follow should help improve children's agility.

Challenge Activities Involving Changes in the Height of the Body

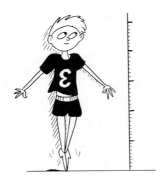

Can you. . .

1. jump as high as you can?
2. jump with as little height as you can?
3. alternate jumping your maximum and minimum?
4. jump as fast as you can?
5. jump as slowly as you can?
6. alternate fast and slow jumping?
7. jump from a full squat?
8. jump as high as you can without using your arms?

9. jump as high as you can while holding an object such as a pillow or beanbag?
10. jump and toss the object to yourself?
11. jump and toss the object to a partner?
12. hop on one foot?
13. hop as high as you can?
14. hop as low as you can?
15. hop four times on one foot and then four times on the other?
16. hop twice on one foot and then twice on the other?
17. alternate hopping once on one foot and then once on the other?
18. bounce on an inner tube as many ways as you can (see the section on challenge activities with inner tubes)?
19. bounce on a trampoline as high as you can?
20. bounce on a trampoline as low as you can?
21. bounce while combining high and low jumping?
22. bounce as high as you can from different leg positions (feet apart, feet together, tuck bounce, pike bounce, and so on)?
23. bounce while using different arm positions (circling, lifting at sides)?
24. coordinate your arms and legs to your bouncing pattern?
25. jump over a stationary rope?
26. jump over a swinging rope?
27. jump over a turning rope?
28. jump over a rope you are turning?
29. jump rope as many ways as you can using different foot patterns?
30. jump rope with a partner?

Challenge Activities Involving Changes in Distance

Can you. . .

1. jump as far as you can?
2. jump as near as you can?
3. jump without using your arms?
4. jump using different arm positions?
5. jump using different leg positions?
6. jump and land with your feet in different positions?
7. land on your toes?
8. land on your heels?
9. land on one foot?
10. land in a squat position?
11. land in a step position?
12. land with your arms at your sides?
13. land with your arms out to your sides?
14. land with your arms overhead?
15. land with your trunk bent in different ways?
16. jump backward?
17. walk backward?

18. run backward or sideward?
19. jump twice, three times, four times?
20. leap over an object?
21. jump off objects?
22. jump and land different ways?
23. jump off objects from different heights?
24. jump off different objects?
25. jump different heights?
26. jump and land on different surfaces?
27. jump and land lightly?
28. jump and continue forward after landing?
29. leap over objects?
30. jump, leap, and change distances as many ways as you can with a partner?

Challenge Activities Involving Changes in Direction

Try to. . .

1. jump and turn (quarter, half, three-quarter, full turn).
2. jump up and change body position (tuck, pike, straddle, stride, and so on).
3. jump up and combine turning with a change in body position, such as a quarter turn with a tuck jump.
4. jump forward, then sideward, and then backward.
5. jump in a circle, square, triangle, and so forth.
6. jump up and land in a different spot.
7. run between chairs.
8. run around a chair.
9. run with many people going in different directions without touching.
10. leap over an object and turn upon landing.
11. jump off objects and turn while in the air.
12. jump off an object and change trunk position in the air.
13. run and jump up onto an object.
14. leap onto an object.
15. run forward and change direction quickly on command.
16. slide sideways and change direction on signal.
17. dodge objects tossed in your direction.
18. move from a high point to a low point and back to a high point as quickly as you can.
19. bounce and turn on an inner tube.
20. bounce and turn on the trampoline.
21. perform stunts on the trampoline (hand and knee drop, knee drop, seat drop, and so on).
22. jump over blocks laid on the ground while moving in different directions.
23. using ropes laid out on the ground, hop or jump from one side to the other.

24. jump over a turning rope and change your body position.
25. jump over a rope you turn and move forward, sideward, or backward.
26. jump over a "poison rope" swung in a circle by a partner.
27. run through a series of tires laid flat on the ground.
28. run around a series of tires placed on the ground.
29. do different stunts around, through, and on a series of tires lying on the ground.
30. do tumbling tricks requiring your body to roll in various ways (log rolls, forward rolls, backward rolls, and so on).
31. do tumbling tricks requiring your body to pass through an inverted support position (cartwheels, round-offs, head springs, back walkovers, front walkovers, and so forth).

FLEXIBILITY

Flexibility, necessary for successful performance in all movement activities, can be defined as the range of motion of a given joint. Most children are very flexible during the preschool and primary grade years. Good flexibility rapidly decreases with age, however, unless one strives to maintain this desirable condition. The following activities are divided into those for improving flexibility in the area of the shoulder girdle and those for improving flexibility in the area of the hip joint. These activities are presented as challenges and incorporate ideas from a variety of activity areas.

Problem-Solving Activities for Shoulder Girdle Flexibility

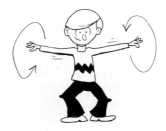

See if you can. . .

1. swing your arms around in a circle vertically, forward and backward.
2. do small arm circles forward or backward with your arms held out to the side.
3. do large arm circles with your arms held out to the side.
4. swing your arms up and back several times.
5. pull your arms back several times from a position of having them outstretched at the side.

6. do the "door opener"; with arms held high, elbows bent, hands next to chin, pull back both arms forcefully several times.
7. place your hands behind your neck and pull your arms back forcefully several times.
8. raise one arm overhead, keeping the other down at your side, and forcefully reverse their positions.
9. do arm circles with your arms extended overhead.
10. reach one hand back over your shoulder and grasp it with the other hand placed behind your back.
11. clasp your hands behind your neck, drop one elbow down, and pull back forcefully.
12. from a position on your stomach with your arms outstretched overhead, lift your head, chest, and arms as high as you can several times.
13. from a position on your stomach, with your fingers interlocked behind your neck, raise your head and chest while forcing your arms backward.
14. from a position on your stomach with your arms extended sideways, move your arms up and down.
15. from the same position as number 14, move your arms in circles.
16. from a position of holding a stick 4 feet long with both hands wide apart, swing it backward and forward over your head.
17. from the same position as number 16, progressively move your hands closer on the stick until they are a shoulder's width apart.
18. from a position of holding the stick overhead with both hands, forcefully move the stick sideways to the left and then to the right.
19. from the same position as number 18, forcefully move the arms backward.
20. swim using the crawl stroke, breast stroke, and back stroke.
21. row a boat.
22. throw a ball.
23. paddle a canoe.
24. climb a ladder.

Problem-Solving Activities for Hip Joint Flexibility

Can you. . .

1. touch your ankles while keeping your legs straight?
2. touch your toes with your feet together?
3. touch your toes with your feet apart?
4. touch your left toe and then your right with your feet apart?
5. touch the floor with your feet in various positions?
6. touch the floor behind you from a straddle position?
7. place your hands behind your neck and bend forward forcefully?
8. place your hands on your hips and bend back forcefully at the waist?
9. combine forceful forward and backward bending?
10. bend sideways from the hip joint?

11. alternate four counts to one side and four counts to the other?
12. alternately bend forward, sideward, and backward at the waist?
13. do continuous trunk circles?
14. from a sitting position with your legs together, bend forward and grasp your ankles?
15. from a sitting position with your legs spread, bend forward and grasp your ankles?
16. from a sitting position with your legs spread, bend forward and grasp one ankle and touch your head to your knee?
17. from the same position as number 16, first touch your left leg, then the floor, and finally your right leg?
18. from a standing position with a long pole resting on your shoulders, turn your trunk first to the left and then to the right?
19. from the same position as number 18, bend sideways at the waist and repeat to the opposite side?
20. with a ball held high over your head, bend forward at the trunk while keeping your arms overhead at all times?
21. from the same position as number 20, bend your trunk first to one side and then to the other?
22. from a position of kneeling on one knee with the opposite leg stretched out to the side, bend to one side and then to the other with your hands on your waist?
23. from the same position as number 22, repeat the activity with your hands and arms in different positions?
24. from the same position as number 22, bend toward the outstretched leg and grasp the toe?
25. from a position of kneeling on both knees with both arms overhead, bend backward at the waist and touch the floor with the hands?
26. repeat number 25, but instead touch the head to the floor?
27. from a sitting position, roll back and touch your toes to the floor?
28. repeat the same action as number 27, keeping the legs straight and together; touch first to your left, then right?
29. practice forward and backward rolls?
30. do a back bridge?
31. do a back bend?

STRENGTH

Strength may be defined simply as the ability to do work against a resistance or heavy load. A necessary factor for success in sports, strength affects the performance quality of many sport activities and of virtually all movement.

The strength of today's North American youth is generally deficient in comparison with boys and girls from several other countries. The primary area of deficiency appears to be in the region of the upper arms and shoulder girdle. Involvement in a variety of hanging, swinging, and climb-

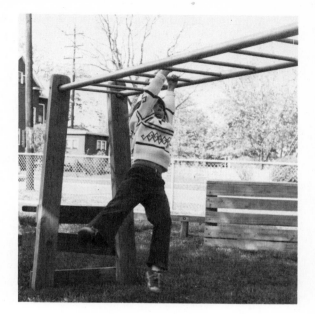

Figure 9–2 The horizontal ladder is excellent for developing shoulder strength. (Courtesy of Creative Playgrounds Corp., Terre Haute, Ind. Used with permission.)

ing activities can do much to improve children's strength in this area of the body (Fig. 9–2).

The following activities for developing strength have been divided into three sections: strength activities for the upper arms and shoulder girdle, strength activities for the abdominal muscles, and strength activities for the legs. Special equipment required for practice in these activities is minimal.

Challenge Activities for Arm and Shoulder Girdle Strength

Can you. . .

1. walk like a bear (on all fours with the arms and legs straight) forward, backward, and sideward?
2. do the "inch worm" (from the push-up position, keep the hands in place, raise the hips, and walk forward until the feet approach the hands; then move hands back out to assume the push-up position again and repeat)?
3. do a mule kick?
4. do a frog hop forward, sideward, and backward?
5. do a puppy run (scamper forward on all fours)?
6. do a lame puppy run (move forward on three body parts)?
7. do a wheelbarrow walk with a partner?
8. do modified push-ups (from knees)?
9. do true push-ups (from toes)?
10. do the crab walk?
11. do the seal walk (a straight body drag)?

12. lie in push-up position and then turn over to your back and back to your front while keeping your body flat at all times?
13. toss and catch a heavy ball (medicine ball) many different ways?
14. support yourself on a climbing rope or pole?
15. support yourself in different ways on the climbing rope?
16. climb a rope or pole?
17. swing from a horizontal bar?
18. swing on a bar and drop off at the end of your swing?
19. travel from one end to the other of a horizontal bar?
20. skin-the-cat on the horizontal bar?
21. crawl on all fours along the underside of the bar?
22. do chin-ups (palms forward)?
23. do pull-ups (palms away)?
24. play tug-of-war?
25. play tug-of-war using a small tire?
26. arm wrestle?
27. wrist wrestle?
28. do a tripod?
29. do a headstand?
30. do a handstand?

Challenge Activities for Abdominal Strength

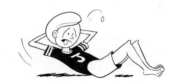

Can you. . .

1. bend forward at the waist and return to an erect position several times?
2. repeat the above activity with the hands and arms progressing from a hands-on-hip position to a position behind the neck and finally to an overhead position?
3. bend forward from the waist several times while holding a ball overhead?
4. from a position on your back and with your arms crossed in front of your chest, raise your head and upper back off the floor and hold for a few seconds?
5. from a position on your back with your knees bent, do sit-ups (arm position should progress from being at sides to in front of stomach to folded in front of chest and finally to folded behind neck)?
6. do sit-ups on an incline?
7. do sit-ups with a weighted object?
8. do sit-ups and twist to the side each time you come up?
9. do single leg raises?

10. do double leg raises?
11. do leg raises and hold?
12. from a sitting position while leaning back on your elbows, raise one leg and hold?
13. same as number 12, but raise both legs?
14. same as number 12, but raise both legs and circle your feet?
15. from a sitting position supported with a straight arm, raise one leg?
16. same as number 15, but raise both legs?
17. same as number 15, but raise both legs to a 45-degree angle and hold?
18. same as number 15, but trace your name with first one foot and then the other?
19. from a sitting position with no hand or arm support, raise one leg and hold?
20. same as number 19, except raise both legs, balance, and hold?

Challenge Activities for Leg Strength

Can you. . .

1. walk up a hill?
2. carry heavy objects?
3. push a heavy object?
4. run as fast as you can?
5. run a long distance?
6. jump as far as you can (broad jump)?
7. jump as high as you can (vertical jump)?
8. do the high jump?
9. run in place?
10. jump rope?
11. ride a tricycle?
12. ride a bicycle?
13. do the runner's sprint start?
14. from a position on your stomach, get to your feet as fast as you can and run to the other end of the room?
15. do same as above, but from a position on your back?
16. do half-squats?
17. do various leg kicks in running?
18. leg wrestle?
19. lunge forward and to the side?
20. lunge backward and to the side?

SUMMARY

We must remember to develop children's physical abilities as well as their movement abilities. Since these two types of abilities are interrelated, many of the activities designed to enhance physical abilities also help develop specific movement abilities and vice versa. Both contribute to a better performance by the child. Therefore, the motor development program should improve children's stability, agility, flexibility, and strength as well as increase their adeptness at performing fundamental movements.

The activities suggested in this chapter are but a sampling of the many possibilities for movement experiences. They may be supplemented and modified in a variety of ways. In selecting a suitable activity, the instructor should be able to answer "yes" to the question, "Will this activity contribute to the child's movement *and* physical abilities?"

BIBLIOGRAPHY

1. Gallahue, David L.: *Motor Development and Movement Experiences for Young Children (3–7).* New York: John Wiley, 1976.
2. Mosston, Muska: *Developmental Movement.* Columbus, Ohio: Charles E. Merrill, 1965.

CHAPTER 10

MOVEMENT EXPERIENCES FOR ENHANCING FUNDAMENTAL LOCOMOTOR ABILITIES

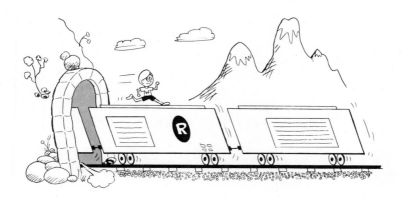

Fundamental locomotor movements enable young children to move through space efficiently and explore their environment. The development of mature locomotor patterns of running and jumping may be considered essential to the refinement of other patterns such as leaping, galloping, hopping, and skipping.

During early childhood, children should have experience in performing all locomotor patterns; when appropriate, indirect teaching approaches should be used. Children over 7 years of age having difficulty with movement should concentrate on refining the basic locomotor patterns of running and jumping before attempting additional movements. These remedial activities for running and jumping should be presented by direct methods to the children. Once the basic patterns of running and jumping are mastered, however, these children may be offered the opportunity to explore more freely the supplemental movements of leaping, galloping, hopping, and skipping.

This chapter contains a list of sample developmental and remedial activities for enhancing the basic locomotor movements of running and jumping. Additional developmental activities for refining the leaping, galloping, hopping, and skipping patterns have been included and are presented in a problem-solving format. The reader is encouraged to develop supplemental activities to improve fundamental locomotor movements.

DEVELOPMENTAL MOVEMENT EXPERIENCES

RUNNING

The development of the running pattern, which has been extensively researched, is detailed in Chapter 3. To encourage development of this pattern, a wide variety of challenge experiences may be incorporated into the motor development program. A list of such activities follows.

Challenge Activities Without Equipment

Can you. . .

1. run forward?
2. run backward?
3. run with your feet wide apart?
4. run with your feet close together?
5. run with your toes out, in, and then forward?
6. run on the sides of your feet?
7. run on your heels or toes?
8. run while crossing one foot over the other?

9. run with your upper body bent forward, sideward, or backward?
10. run with your knees high?
11. run and swing your arms in different ways?
12. run with your arms above your head, to the side, and so on?
13. run with your body stretched high?
14. run with your body held at a high level?
15. run with your body held at a low level?
16. run and touch the ground, alternating hands?
17. run in a low position, touching the ground with both hands as you go?
18. run at different speeds?
19. run to a musical beat?
20. run fast or slowly with short and then long strides?
21. run in place?
22. run while shuffling your feet?
23. run with long strides?
24. run and shift your weight from side to side?
25. run in a straight, angular, or zigzag pattern or some other geometric shape or design?
26. run and weave between, around, or through obstacles?
27. run letter or number patterns?
28. run while looking over your right, then left, shoulder?
29. run as lightly or quietly as possible?
30. run with heavy or hard steps?
31. bounce as high as you can while you run?
32. run like a wooden soldier?
33. run like a rag doll?
34. run up and down the stairs or bleachers?
35. run through an obstacle course?
36. run like a camel, giraffe, horse, and so on?
37. run like your mother, your father, a clown, and so forth?
38. pretend you are running on ice or in snow, sand, mud, and so on?
39. pretend you are running uphill, downhill, or on the side of a hill?
40. pretend you are running against or with a strong wind?
41. run as many different ways as possible with a partner?
42. avoid bumping into people while running?
43. run and stop when I clap once?
44. pick one place in the room and then run to it and back without touching anyone?
45. run as quietly as you can?
46. start in a very low position and go to the highest running position?
47. run in slow motion?
48. run around and between objects in the room?
49. run like an animal that runs quickly?
50. run like a character you have seen on television?

51. pretend you are running at the beach?
52. pretend you are running in the rain?

Problem-Solving Activities with Equipment (Hoops)

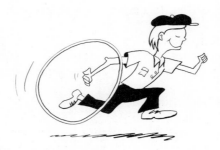

Can you. . .

1. run with the hoop in many ways?
2. run around a hoop that is lying on the floor?
3. balance the hoop and run around it while holding with one hand?
4. run around a vertically balanced hoop?
5. roll the hoop and run around it?
6. roll the hoop and run with it?
7. run faster than a rolling hoop?
8. toss the hoop, run, and then catch it before it touches the ground?
9. do a fast zigzag run between several hoops?
10. run through a line of hoops without touching them?
11. run while tossing and catching a hoop?
12. roll a hoop and keep it going with a stick while running alongside it?
13. run under a hoop held by a partner?
14. run through a hoop rolled by a partner?
15. and your partner get through a rolling hoop before it stops?
16. and your partner run alongside each other while tossing and catching hoops?

Problem-Solving Activities with Partners

Can you. . .

1. find several ways to run with a partner?
2. run around the room without touching anyone?
3. run across the room without touching anyone?

4. run alongside a partner?
5. run behind a partner without touching him?
6. run while holding hands with a partner?
7. run and change direction on command without touching anyone?
8. run and return to your space on command?
9. run backward with your partner?
10. run while facing your partner?

JUMPING

The development of the jumping pattern distance, which was discussed in detail in Chapter 3, may be promoted by incorporation of a wide variety of challenging and fun problem-solving experiences into the developmental program. The following list of movement experiences are designed to encourage refinement of the jumping pattern.

Challenge Activities Without Equipment

Can you. . .

1. jump as far as possible?
2. jump with lightness? Can you be light and airy like a feather while you jump?
3. stretch when you jump? Stretch one body part and then two and three while you jump.
4. express smoothness while you jump? Can you express smoothness with your arms while jumping?
5. stay low to the floor and still be jumping?
6. jump like a popcorn kernel popping? How explosively can you jump?
7. jump up like a rocket?
8. jump forward? sidewards? backward?
9. jump off and on one foot in as many ways as possible?
10. jump with your feet close together?
11. jump with your legs far apart in stride position?
12. jump and do a quarter turn, half turn, and full turn?
13. find many different ways to twist your body while jumping?
14. jump as long as possible?
15. jump with short jumps?
16. jump like a rabbit or a kangaroo?
17. jump up and down and stay in your place on the floor using one foot? Left foot? Right foot? Both feet?
18. jump while making a circle over your head with your arms? In front of your body?
19. find many different ways to move your hands when you jump?
20. bend your body in many different ways when you jump?
21. move your legs when you jump?
22. move your arms when you jump?

23. touch your legs with your hands when jumping?
24. jump in different ways around the room?
25. jump in different directions?
26. jump as far as you can?
27. jump in place but at different speeds?
28. jump and turn your body in the air?
29. jump and move your legs in the air?
30. jump with your legs crossed?
31. jump with one foot forward and one backward?
32. jump with one arm forward and one backward?
33. jump and land lightly? On what part of your foot did you land?
34. jump and land heavily? On what part of your foot did you land this time?
35. jump as high as you can? Try again to go higher. How do you start when you want to go higher?
36. jump and reach out?
37. jump and reach up?
38. jump backward without jumping into someone?

Challenge Activities with Equipment (Short Ropes, Balls, Hoops, Blocks, Boards, Maps)

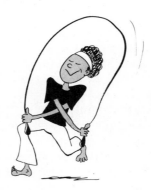

Can you. . .

1. do different things with your rope?
2. move the rope back and forth and jump over it?
3. move the rope around your partner's body with one hand while jumping in different forms? With the other hand? Over your head? On your left side? Right side?
4. jump over a rope lying on the floor?

5. make a circle with your partner's rope and jump into the center and out again?
6. jump sideways (backward, and so on) over two parallel ropes?
7. alternately jump long and short distances alongside a rope?
8. jump back and forth across the ropes?
9. alternately jump from one side of the rope to the other?
10. find ways of combining jumping with different locomotor movements using the ropes?
11. jump over one rope and go under a second?
12. find different ways to jump over two ropes lying on the floor?
13. jump from rope to rope stretched out on the ground?
14. jump over two parallel ropes lying on the floor?
15. jump over two ropes spread out on the floor?
16. jump as far as you can and measure with the rope?
17. find different ways to jump over a suspended rope?
18. jump from one end of the line of fire to the other?
19. move the rope under your feet using just one hand?
20. turn the rope and jump over it?
21. turn the rope, jump over it, and move around the floor?
22. turn the rope in a different direction and jump over it?
23. jump with both feet at the same time?
24. hop over the rope while it is turning?
25. hop on alternate feet while the rope is turning?
26. combine the jump and the hop while you are turning the rope?
27. cross your arms and still continue to jump rope?
28. jump more than once between turns of the rope?
29. lay your rope stretched out on the ground and jump over it?
30. jump from one end of the rope to the other end of the rope?
31. get over the rope as you are swinging it on the floor?
32. jump slowly with the rope?
33. move around the room jumping rope? Hopping on one or both feet? Skipping fast or slowly?
34. jump and bounce a ball? Bounce close to the ground? Bounce using high bounces?
35. bounce the ball, jump and turn, and continue bouncing the ball?
36. jump in and out of the hoops? Use as many different body shapes as you can.
37. start out running and jump over the block?
38. jump off the block and land with both feet in stride position? With both feet together?
39. do different arm movements while jumping off the block? Do different leg movements?
40. jump off the block and keep your knees stiff? Bent slightly? Bent all the way in squat position? Try all of these. Which one do you like best?
41. jump the word "cat," and so forth, using an alphabet board?

42. jump from the Ohio River to the Gulf of Mexico using the map of the United States?

Challenge Activities with Partners and Long Ropes

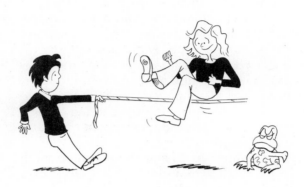

Use a long stationary rope held a few inches above the ground by two people.

Who can. . .

1. find different ways to get over the rope?
2. jump over the rope?
3. jump in a different direction over the rope?
4. jump as high as they can over the rope?
5. jump as low as they can over the rope?
6. jump as far as they can over the rope?
7. jump as softly as they can?
8. jump as big as they can?
9. jump as small as they can?
10. jump over with a partner?
11. find different ways to jump with a partner?
12. jump over and back?
13. jump over and back with a partner?
14. repeat the above challenges with a rope swung like a pendulum?
15. jump over a twining rope?
16. find the most ways to jump over a turning rope?
17. run in through a turning rope and out the other side?
18. run in, jump, and run out of a turning rope?
19. jump over a turning rope_____times (1, 2, 3, and so on)?
20. turn around while jumping over a turning rope?

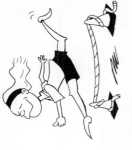

REMEDIAL MOVEMENT EXPERIENCES

Running

The following remedial movement experiences are designed to enhance specific components of the running pattern. The instructor should especially concentrate on having the children develop an efficient leg and arm action.

POINTS TO EMPHASIZE

Complete leg extension, increased leg action, balanced position.

MOVEMENT EXPERIENCES

Rope Run

Place a series of short ropes on the ground or floor and instruct the children to run perpendicular to them, taking one step between each rope. As the children become proficient at running the ropes, increase the space between each rope. This will force the children to increase both their stride length and the duration of flight.

ADAPTATIONS

1. Vary the amount of space between the ropes and have the children run, adjusting their stride to the various changes in distance between ropes.
2. Have the children run while holding their arms in various positions. What happens?
3. Have the children run backward through the rope course.
4. Have the children run first on their toes, then on their heels, and finally flatfootedly.

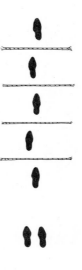

POINTS TO EMPHASIZE

Utilize the arms to maintain stability; legs should move rapidly.

MOVEMENT EXPERIENCES

Obstacle Course

Place cones, hoops, or chairs in various patterns on the floor. Have the children attempt to run through each course by using a controlled running pattern. The following are examples of various patterns that can be constructed with cones.

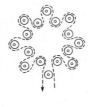

ADAPTATIONS

1. Vary the spacing between the cones, hoops, or chairs, and vary the patterns to include stopping, starting, running in circles, and so on.
2. Have the children attempt to run through the obstacle course while holding their arms in various positions. What role do the arms play?

Control run; lift leg high; time jump; maintain balance; utilize arms; extend legs completely.

Modified Hurdle Run

Construct hurdles by using cones or chairs and rope. Suspend the rope between the cones and thread the rope into the top of each cone or over the leg braces of the chairs. Leave at least one end of each rope free so that if it is kicked or hit it will not trip the runner.

Initially suspend the ropes loosely between cones so that they can be cleared easily. Place the hurdles far apart so that children have sufficient time to prepare for each hurdle.

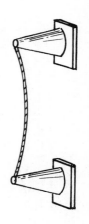

1. Gradually tighten the suspended ropes, thereby increasing the leg lift needed to successfully clear the rope.
2. Vary the distance between each cone, thus increasing the difficulty of the run.
3. Vary the pattern in which the cones are laid out, thereby forcing the children to adjust their running pattern, raise their legs higher, and lead with both the dominant and non-dominant foot.

POINTS TO EMPHASIZE	MOVEMENT EXPERIENCES	ADAPTATIONS

Legs swing from the hip; arms swing in a vertical plane.

Line Running

Have the children run along various types of lines that have been marked on the floor. The children should attempt to make foot contact on the line as their leg swings straight through to heel strike. Initially have the children run a straight line and with success progress to a large circle, smaller circle, and curved path.

1. Add a second line that runs parallel to the first approximately 1 foot from it. Have the children make contact between the lines as they run. With success, decrease the distance between lines.
2. Have the children attempt to run without using their arms. What happens?
3. Tell the children to run fast, slowly, forward, backward, and so on.

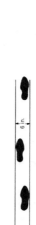

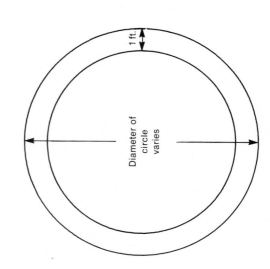

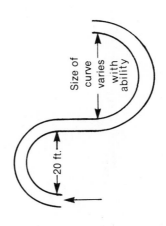

POINTS TO EMPHASIZE

Complete leg extension, good flight, coordinated arm swing, controlled run.

MOVEMENT EXPERIENCES

Hoop Running

Place hoops in various patterns on the floor and have the children attempt to make foot contact in each hoop as they run. The following are examples of various patterns that can be utilized.

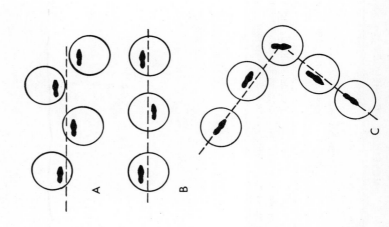

ADAPTATIONS

1. Vary the patterns, but be sure you run the hoop patterns yourself so that you know their level of difficulty.
2. Increase the distance between the hoops, thereby forcing the children to increase both leg stride and duration of flight (Fig. 10–6).

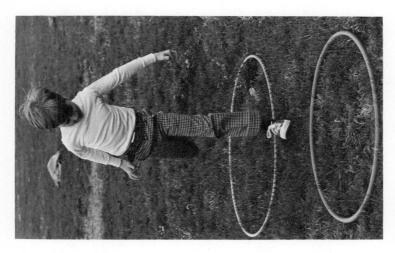

Figure 10–1 Running in hoops can aid in lengthening stride and increasing duration of flight.

Arms are bent at right angles, and they swing from the shoulder in a vertical plane.

Arm Weight

Have the children hold objects of equal weight in each hand. The objects should be small enough to be easily held and should weigh under one pound; a tennis ball with shot would work well. The children should attempt to run while holding these objects.

1. Have the children run and swing the arms in various ways and explore how the arm action affects the leg action.
2. Vary the weight of the objects.
3. Have the children run and rapidly change direction. What role do the arms play?

Jumping

The following remedial experiences are designed to enhance specific body actions of the jumping pattern. Children having difficulty with the jumping pattern should be provided with experiences to develop arm, trunk, and leg-hip movements.

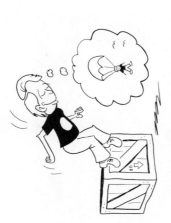

POINTS TO EMPHASIZE

Eyes straight ahead for stability, synchronized arm swirl at takeoff, stable flight, foot position at landing for stability, efficient absorption of momentum at landing.

MOVEMENT EXPERIENCES

Parachute Jump

Have the children stand on a raised platform, pile of mats, or sturdy chair and jump onto a mat that has been placed on the floor. The children should be allowed to choose any of several heights from which to jump. The children should attempt to use both feet at takeoff and landing. Children who have difficulty in jumping simultaneously with both feet should jump from a lower height. The arms should move upward in synchronization during the preparatory phase and should be held outward for increased stability during flight and landing. The feet should be approximately shoulder width apart at landing, and the legs should absorb the body's downward momentum.

ADAPTATIONS

1. Have the children jump with the arms and feet in various positions.
2. Ask the children to jump forward, sideward, and backward and explore what is done differently with each jump.
3. Have the children attempt to twist a quarter, half, or full turn while jumping. Concentrate on good form.
4. Have the children jump from various heights and upon landing perform various self-testing stunts, forward and backward rolls, frog stand, head stand, and so on.

POINTS TO EMPHASIZE	MOVEMENT EXPERIENCES	ADAPTATIONS

ADAPTATIONS

Blast Off

Good leg crouch, rapid arm swing, reach at landing, explosive leg action, efficient absorption of force at landing.

Have each child find a space on the floor, or have each child stand in a hoop that has been previously placed around the room. As the instructor and children count down from 10, the children should slowly increase their leg crouch. At zero count, or "blast off," the children should attempt to jump as high as possible in a vertical direction.

1. Explore with the children how the arms play a role in the jumping action. Try jumping while holding the arms in various positions.

2. Have the children attempt to jump and mark a piece of paper that has been taped to the wall.

3. Instruct the children to work in pairs and attempt to jump beside a wall that has been marked in inches. As one child jumps, the other should observe the height of the jump. Encourage the children to explore various patterns of jumping to find out which is most efficient.

4. Have the children jump and attempt to twist quarter, half, three-quarter, and full turns while in the air. They should work on acquiring good form and a stable landing.

5. Have children toss a large ball in the air and attempt to catch it at the height of their jump.

Rope Jump

Leg extension, arm swirl, legs pulled upward after takeoff.

Suspend a piece of rope from two cones, chairs, or boxes. Have children stand behind the rope and attempt to jump to the other side using both feet simultaneously in takeoff and landing. Initially the rope should be close to the ground, and with successful performance by the children its height can be increased.

1. Have the children jump the rope with the arms held in various positions.

2. Have the children attempt to jump over the rope forward, backward, and sideward.

3. Instruct the children to jump the rope rhythmically forward, backward, and sideward. Develop patterns and program them to various rhythms or music.

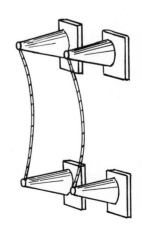

POINTS TO EMPHASIZE	MOVEMENT EXPERIENCES	ADAPTATIONS

River Jump

Both feet used in takeoff and landing, efficient arm swirl, forward lean at takeoff.

The children should find a space on the ground or floor and extend two short ropes alongside each other at their feet. They should then jump over the ropes using both feet simultaneously in takeoff and landing. After each successful attempt at jumping the ropes, the children should increase the distance between the ropes.

1. Explore with the children various other ways to get across the ropes.
2. Have the children jump with the arms held in various positions—behind their backs, over their heads, and so on. What happens to their jumping ability?
3. Tell the children to jump the ropes forward, backward, or sideward. What do they have to do differently?

Target Jump

Flexion at the hips during flight, rapid arm swing, stable flight and landing.

Divide the class into small groups of approximately 3 children each. Supply each group with two cones or chairs, a short piece of rope (jump rope size), and a hoop. Have each group set up the following jump with obstacles:

1. Have the children explore various methods of jumping, including a 2 foot takeoff and landing, a 1 foot takeoff and landing, a 2 foot takeoff and 1 foot landing, and a 1 foot take-off and 2 foot landing.
2. Have the children attempt to jump from a forward, backward, and sideward direction and land in the hoop. Observe how they have to adjust their movements.
3. Have the children jump first with straight legs and then with the legs pulled up tight. Which is more efficient? Why?

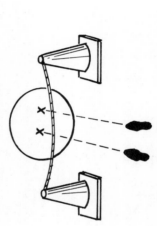

The children should initially attempt to jump over a low rope and land in the hoop using both feet in takeoff and landing. As the children improve, they may raise the rope as well as move the hoop farther away from the rope.

POINTS TO EMPHASIZE

A well-timed jumping action, arms held outward to maintain balance during flight, explosive takeoff, balanced landing.

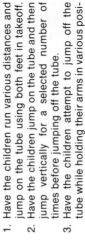

MOVEMENT EXPERIENCES

Tube Jump

Make several inner tube trampolines. The class should be divided into several small groups, each with its own trampoline. Each child should take turns jumping onto the trampoline and jumping off in propelled flight. Explore with the children various types of jumps: those on two feet, or one foot; those with arms held in various positions, and so on.

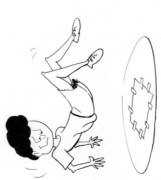

ADAPTATIONS

1. Have the children run various distances and jump on the tube using both feet in takeoff.
2. Have the children jump on the tube and then jump vertically for a selected number of times before jumping off the tube.
3. Have the children attempt to jump off the tube while holding their arms in various positions.

MOVEMENT EXPERIENCES DESIGNED TO ENHANCE SUPPLEMENTAL LOCOMOTOR PATTERNS

LEAPING

Leaping, which is actually an exaggerated run with a longer flight phase, is usually combined with running because it is difficult to sustain the pattern by itself. There has been little research on the development of the leaping pattern. A list of challenge experiences that involve leaping follows.

See if you can. . .

1. run several steps and leap.
2. leap in place.
3. leap to a specific point and return to the original position.
4. find two spots away from your "home" spot, leap to one spot and then the other, and return "home" as quickly as possible.
5. perform a continuous series of leaps for distance and not for height.
6. take the fewest leaps to get across the center line.
7. leap a distance between two lines. Do a series of leaps without running steps between them; emphasize distance and height in the leap.
8. take a run-run-leap, run-run-leap from here to there (or around the area). Then take a leap-leap-jump, leap-leap-jump.
9. while standing in a circle with other children, leap a set of steps in one direction.
10. stand in a big circle with one of you in the middle. Sometimes leap toward the person in the center and sometimes leap away from the person.
11. leap to a target or series of target areas.
12. leap and stop on signal. See how quickly you can stop on signal.
13. leap on the "pop" in "Pop Goes the Weasel."
14. leap from a slow and then a fast run.
15. combine leaps with one or more steps in patterns such as step-leap or step-leap-leap.
16. combine two running steps and a leap, at first giving all three steps the same time value of the run. Make the leaps as high as possible.
17. leap among classmates within a large area while avoiding contact. Repeat, reducing the area as much as you can.
18. lift your arms as high as possible at the height of the leap. Leap with the same arm and leg forward. Leap with the opposite arm and leg forward. Which way is more comfortable?
19. perform a series of running leaps while keeping the arms stiff.
20. move your legs, arms, and trunk into various positions during the flight phase of the leap.
21. place masking tape X's on the floor. Leap from X to X. Weave in and around them.

22. leap in a circle (square, triangle, and so on) while moving from one point to another.
23. draw a pattern of many connected straight lines on a large piece of paper and leap that pattern. Now leap a pattern first and then draw it on a large piece of paper.
24. leap in the pattern of a "C" or "Z". Can you leap the pattern of the first letter in your first name? Can you spell your whole first name by leaping? What other words can you spell by leaping?
25. while leaping different floor patterns, make patterns in the air with your head and arms. While leaping a floor pattern, make different patterns in the air with a ball large enough for both hands to clutch.
26. arrange stepping stones around the floor and leap from one to the next.
27. leap from letter to letter taped on the floor.
28. find a partner close to you. You and your partner put your ropes together on the floor in an interesting pattern and leap over and around the ropes in time to a beat.
29. stretch a rope out on the floor. How would a rabbit, a deer, and so on get over it? Leap over an obstacle course of scattered ropes on the floor. Leap around the room while swinging a rope?
30. leap over a rope on the floor (raise the rope off the floor gradually).
31. leap into the air as high as you can. Do it on the other foot. What do you do before you leap?
32. take a short leap. How did you land?
33. run and take a long leap. What sport skill is something like this? How is it different from a run? How is it like a run?
34. leap in motion.
35. leap and move another part of your body.
36. leap to the side.
37. leap across two ropes (or lines) on the floor.
38. leap over an object.
39. leap and throw or catch a ball.
40. run-run-leap and repeat several times, leading first with one foot and then with the other.

GALLOPING

Galloping, a favorite movement pattern of young children, is used in a variety of games and activities involving imagination. Unfortunately, there is almost no information about the development of the galloping pattern. It may be acquired after the walking and running patterns have been established, as it is a combination of the two. In the gallop, one foot leads throughout; the other foot is rapidly brought up to it, and the lead foot again extends. These movements should be smooth and rhythmical. The arms may be lifted or held down at the sides.

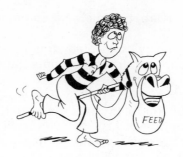

Can you. . .

1. move forward and keep one foot in front of the other all the time? How high can you gallop? How smoothly can you gallop? Can you gallop smoothly, turning in one place?
2. gallop lightly forward and then make one high galloping step?
3. gallop with a big lift?
4. pretend you're a big horse galloping?
5. gallop lightly like a small pony? Good percussion instruments to use are coconut shells, wood blocks, and claves.
6. gallop among classmates within a large area, avoiding personal contact? Repeat, narrowing the area as much as possible.
7. gallop to a specific point and return to the original position?
8. find two spots away from your "home" spot, gallop to one spot and then the other, and return "home" as quickly as possible?
9. on the signal, change your level of height? Change level and direction while galloping. Keep hands low while galloping at a high level. Keep hands high while galloping at a low level. Can you change levels while galloping but keep one part of the body at a constant level?
10. scatter around the room and then travel with quick gallops toward the center of the room and hold your position? Slowly rise to a high level and then sink to a low one. Go back to your starting place with quick, lively galloping steps.
11. gallop a set number of times in one direction and then change direction while in a circle with other children?
12. gallop to a target or series of target areas in some geometric shape?
13. stand in a big circle with one of you in the middle and then sometimes gallop towards the person in the center and sometimes gallop away from the person in the center?
14. gallop as many places as you can, changing directions as you go? See how quickly you can change direction. Change directions every time you hear a signal change.
15. see how slowly you can gallop while staying in your own area? Now see how quietly and quickly you can gallop. Now follow the

sound of the drum beats or hand claps. When they go faster, you move faster. When they slow down, you move more slowly.

16. gallop to the pulse beat you set yourself? You may make clicks or pops with your mouth, or you may clap a hand on your body. Change the tempo of your beat.

17. gallop slowly without much lift?

18. gallop and stop on signal? See how quickly you can stop on signal.

19. gallop along different pathways? There are two main pathways you can make: curved or straight. If you put two straight pathways together with sharp corners you can make a zigzag path. How many pathways can you devise?

20. and a partner put your ropes together on the floor in an interesting pattern and gallop over and around the ropes in time to a beat?

21. gallop in a circle, square, and so on, while moving from one point to another?

22. draw a pattern on a large piece of paper and gallop that pattern? Now gallop a pattern first and then draw it on a large piece of paper.

23. gallop in the pattern of a "C" or "Z"? Can you gallop the pattern of the first letter of your first name?

24. make patterns in the air with your hands and arms while galloping different floor patterns? While galloping a floor pattern, make different patterns in the air with a ball large enough for both hands to clutch.

25. scatter ropes in an obstacle course on the floor and gallop around or between them?

26. make a pathway with your ropes to and away from a box? Gallop down the pathway, leap over the box, and continue galloping down the pathway.

27. make geometric patterns with beanbags, chairs, hoops, and so on. Have the children gallop between them.

28. tape letters on the floor and gallop from letter to letter, spelling out words?

29. gallop while holding hands with a partner?

30. gallop around a stationary partner, and then exchange places?

31. keep your arms low while galloping?

32. keep your arms high while galloping?

33. gallop fast and gallop slow?

34. gallop high and gallop low?

35. gallop sideways and backward? Which is easiest? Why?

36. gallop with a partner?

37. gallop in circles?

38. gallop like a horse?

39. gallop in a different way?

40. gallop and move in other ways with a partner?

HOPPING

Hopping is an interesting movement pattern to observe in children because of the experimental nature of its development. The hop should be performed rhythmically with an upward or forward thrust, with takeoff and landing occurring on the same foot. On the takeoff, the toes of the thrusting foot leave the ground last. They are first to touch on landing, followed by the ball of the foot and then the heel. The arms are used simultaneously in an upward or forward thrust. There has been little research on the acquisition of the hopping pattern, but it is safe to assume that it begins to develop along with jumping and precedes skipping.

The following list is a compilation of various challenge activities involving hopping. They may prove effective in refining the mature rhythmical hopping pattern.

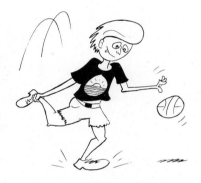

Can you try to. . .

1. hop on your right foot?
2. hop on your left foot?
3. hop forward by alternating your right and left feet?
4. hop backward?
5. hop forward halfway to the wall and backward the rest of the way?
6. hop backward halfway to the wall and forward the rest of the way? Do the same using both feet.
7. hop as lightly as possible?
8. hop with tiny, fast steps?
9. hop with giant hops?
10. hop forward three times on one foot and then backward on the other foot?
11. bounce as high as possible while hopping? Gradually reduce the height.
12. hop low and then gradually increase the height?
13. hop low while touching the ground on either side with one hand?
14. hop low while touching the ground on both sides simultaneously?
15. hop slowly and then suddenly change to a fast pace?

16. hop fast and then suddenly change to a slow pace?
17. hop in a zigzag pattern, changing directions every few steps?
18. hop while tracing different patterns on the floor: squares, triangles, and so on?
19. hop over any object in the room?
20. hop while holding on to something stationary in the room?
21. hop while reaching as high as possible with both hands?
22. hop and move your arms in different ways?
23. hop with no arm movement?
24. hop with various arm swing movements?
25. hop and clap hands on the beat?
26. hop and clap hands off the beat?
27. hop with the nonsupport leg backward, forward, and sideward?
28. hop on your left foot while your right hand holds on to your right leg, or the nonsupport leg?
29. hop on your right foot while your left hand holds on to your left leg, or the nonsupport leg?
30. hop and turn at the same time?
31. hop with your eyes closed?
32. hop while moving away from me and keeping your eyes on me at the same time?
33. hop on your toes?
34. hop but only move certain parts of your body, such as head, trunk, and so on?
35. hop and carry a beanbag on your free foot?
36. hop and toss a beanbag up to your hands with your free foot?
37. hop like an Indian doing a rain dance?
38. hop and bounce a ball? In place? Moving?
39. hop and bounce a ball under the nonsupport leg?
40. throw and catch a ball or beanbag while hopping?
41. balance the beanbag on your head while hopping? Balance it on other body parts?
42. hop over or through a hoop?
43. hop over a wand held at different levels?
44. hop as many ways as you can with your beanbag or ball?
45. hop from side to side over a rope?

SKIPPING

Skipping is a complex movement pattern in which the two sides of the body alternate moving rhythmically. Each leg must coordinate a series of steps and hops at a relatively rapid pace with good knee lift, while the arms simultaneously work rhythmically opposite the action of the legs. Skipping itself has little real value in specific sport skill development. It is, however, an excellent movement pattern for developing coordination between both sides of the body. Little is known about the development of the skipping pattern, but it generally appears to be the last locomotor movement pattern to mature. A list of several challenge activities involving skipping follows.

Let's see if you can. . .

1. skip as many ways as possible.
2. skip forward.
3. skip backward.
4. skip forward halfway to the wall and backward the rest of the way.
5. skip backward halfway to the wall and forward the rest of the way.
6. skip as lightly as possible.
7. skip with giant strides.
8. skip as high as possible while moving. Gradually reduce the height.
9. skip low and then gradually increase the height.
10. skip low, touching the ground on either side with one hand.
11. skip low, touching the ground with both hands simultaneously.
12. skip slowly and then suddenly change to a fast pace.
13. skip fast and then suddenly change to a slow pace.
14. skip in a zigzag pattern, and changing directions every few steps.
15. skip while tracing different patterns on the floor: squares, triangles, and so on.
16. skip while reaching as high as possible with both hands.
17. skip and move your arms in different ways.
18. skip with no arm movement.
19. skip with different arm swing movements.
20. skip and clap hands on the beat.
21. skip and clap hands off the beat.
22. skip and turn at the same time.
23. skip with your eyes closed.
24. skip while looking at me and moving away from me at the same time.
25. skip on your toes.
26. skip but move only certain parts of your body, such as head, trunk, and so on.
27. skip as many ways as you can with a ball or beanbag.
28. skip and bounce a ball at the same time.
29. skip in different ways with a partner.
30. skip with a partner to the music.
31. step and hop on one foot. Change feet. What movement have you discovered?
32. try skipping in different directions.
33. skip sideward in both directions. How did your feet cross? Can you make them do it a different way?
34. skip in a shape. What shape did you make? How many skips did it take you?
35. skip high and skip low.
36. skip fast and skip slowly.
37. skip and bounce a ball.

38. skip and jump rope.
39. skip high. Look at your arms. How did you make yourself skip higher?
40. skip fast. This time use tiny steps, but keep going fast.
41. skip slowly. Use giant skips. When might you skip this way?
42. skip with your arms above your head.
43. skip with your arms at your side.
44. skip with your arms moving. Which is the easiest way of all? How does this way help you skip?
45. skip with a partner.
46. try some other movements while you are skipping.

SUMMARY

This chapter has presented a wide variety of sample developmental and remedial activities suitable for improving fundamental locomotor abilities. The instructor should modify these activities and design new movement experiences to satisfy the psychomotor needs of the particular children being dealt with.

BIBLIOGRAPHY

1. Dauer, Victor P., and Pangrazi, Robert P.: *Dynamic Physical Education for Elementary School Children.* Minneapolis: Burgess, 1975.
2. Gallahue, David L.: *Motor Development and Movement Experiences for Young Children (3–7).* New York: John Wiley, 1976.
3. Gallahue, David L., Werner, Peter H., and Luedke, George C.: *A Conceptual Approach to Moving and Learning.* New York: John Wiley, 1975.
4. Schurr, Evelyn: *Movement Experiences for Children.* Englewood Cliffs, N.J.: Prentice-Hall, 1975.
5. Vannier, MaryHelen, and Gallahue, David L.: *Teaching Physical Education in Elementary Schools.* Philadelphia: W. B. Saunders Co., 1978.

CHAPTER 11

MOVEMENT EXPERIENCES FOR ENHANCING FUNDAMENTAL MANIPULATIVE ABILITIES

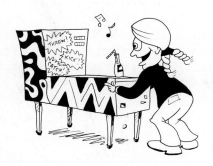

Fundamental manipulative patterns involve use of the extremities in propelling, controlling, or receiving force from an object. This chapter has been structured in a fashion similar to the previous chapter dealing with locomotor patterns. Developmental and remedial activities for the basic patterns of throwing, catching, and kicking have been provided. Movement experiences of a more indirect type for the rolling, bouncing, and striking patterns have also been included. The reader is encouraged to develop additional experiences for these and other movement patterns.

DEVELOPMENTAL MOVEMENT EXPERIENCES

THROWING

Throwing, the first pattern involving propulsion that the young child develops, is dependent upon practice for mature development. The throwing pattern is described in detail in Chapter 4. The throw may be performed in an underhand, overhand, or sidearm manner and may be varied in a great many ways, depending upon the size of the object to be thrown and the orientation of the performer. The following throwing activities may be considered both developmental and remedial in nature.

Challenge Activities to Develop Underhand Throwing Abilities

Using a large ball (an 8½-inch playground ball), can you . . .

1. throw with the feet wide apart and then close together?
2. throw with one foot in front of the other and the feet close or wide apart?
3. throw from a position of sitting on heels or of kneeling on both knees or one knee?
4. throw, varying the degree of body lean forward and sideward?
5. throw, varying the degree of knee and hip flexion?
6. throw with the arms bent slightly and fully extended?
7. throw as slowly or as quickly as you can?
8. throw as easily or as hard as you can?
9. throw with rigid or loose form?
10. throw to the rhythm of a verbal cue, hand clap, drum beat, or music?
11. throw while moving the arms in a small, medium, or large arc?
12. throw with the arm swing as low or as high as possible?
13. throw at a low, medium (chest high), or high target?
14. throw, emphasizing follow-through, at low, medium, or high targets?
15. vary targets so that the throws require different arcs?
16. throw the ball so that it lands between two ropes?
17. throw the ball so that it lands in a hoop or a circled rope?
18. throw the ball into a box, through the back of a chair, onto a chair seat, over a balance beam, or at an Indian club?

19. walk, hop, or jump and then throw at a target?
20. throw at a moving target, such as a rolled inner tube, tire, or cage-ball?
21. throw the ball against a wall?
22. carry the ball and climb onto a vaulting stand, throw to a target, jump off, and skip to retrieve it?
23. throw and catch with a partner on the floor, on a bench, or on a balance beam?
24. push the ball upward from chest level by placing the hands slightly behind and below the ball?
25. use the right or left hand to toss the ball above the head?
26. throw the ball as slowly, as quickly, as easily, as hard, as high, or as low as possible?
27. toss the ball overhead and let it bounce before catching it?
28. toss the ball through or into an overhead target such as a hula hoop?
29. do a vertical toss while walking on the floor, a bench, or a low balance beam?
30. toss the ball up (high or low), clap the hands, let the ball bounce, and then catch it?
31. throw as if you are putting the ball in orbit?

Using a small ball or beanbag, can you . . .

32. balance on one foot (same foot as throwing arm), swing the throwing arm forward, and stride with the nonsupport leg? Repeat this drill, emphasizing rhythm and the length of the stride.
33. throw at targets from a position of sitting or of kneeling on both knees or one knee from different distances and heights (body support, range, level, and direction)?
34. throw as hard, easily, quickly or slowly as you can?
35. walk, run, jump, or hop and throw the ball or beanbag at a target?
36. throw at a moving target?
37. make variations using first the right hand, then the left, emphasizing coordination of both sides of the body?
38. balance the ball or beanbag on one hand and toss it back and forth from one hand to the other?
39. throw different types of balls?
40. throw in different directions?
41. throw at different levels?
42. throw at different speeds?
43. throw like a robot?
44. throw like a rag doll?
45. throw from different body positions?
46. find as many ways as you can to throw underhand?
47. throw to a partner?
48. throw at a target?
49. throw to a moving person?

50. throw at a moving target?
51. toss the ball or beanbag and make it bounce once before hitting a target area?

Challenge Activities to Develop Overhand Throwing Activities

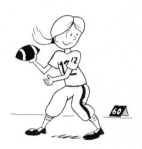

Can you . . .

1. throw a small ball with the feet close together or wide apart and in a normal or stride stance?
2. throw from various bases of support, such as sitting or kneeling?
3. with the arm up close to the ear and the elbow flexed, throw and extend the hand toward a target?
4. throw with the arm slightly bent or fully extended in an overhead or sidearm pattern?
5. throw an object across the front of the body at a target?
6. throw, varying the degree of body lean forward and sideward?
7. with an overhand pattern involving both arms, throw an object at a target?
8. pretend to throw a ball over a tall tree, a wide river, a low fence, or into a mud puddle?
9. run and throw an object at a target?
10. throw an object at a moving target, such as an old tire or cageball?
11. throw an object at a target and hop, skip, run, or crawl to retrieve your object?
12. throw a small, large, heavy, or light object as slowly or as quickly as you can?
13. use a long stride and reach to throw an object at a target?
14. accent the coordination of the arm movement and leg stride in throwing at a target by using a verbal cue, hand clap, or drum beat?
15. throw while moving the arm in a small, medium, or large arc?
16. throw to a low, medium (chest high), or high target?

17. vary the target challenges so that throws require different arcs?
18. throw hard?
19. throw easily?
20. throw fast?
21. throw slowly?
22. throw the ball far?
23. throw with your feet together?
24. throw with your feet apart?
25. throw while standing on one foot?
26. throw with your right, then left, foot forward? Which way works best?
27. throw while facing your target?
28. throw with your side to the target? Which is best?
29. throw with your legs straight?
30. throw with some knee bend? Which is best?
31. throw with no follow-through?
32. throw with follow-through? Which is best?
33. throw to a partner?
34. throw at a target?
35. throw to a moving person?
36. throw at a moving target?
37. throw over a bar or rope?
38. throw over a suspended rope at a target or to a person?

CATCHING

Catching is another manipulative pattern requiring practice for complete development. A detailed review of the basic catching patterns is presented in Chapter 4. A list of developmental and remedial catching activities that also involve throwing follows. Balls of different sizes and other objects may be used for these activities.

Challenge Activities with Large Balls

Can you . . .

1. catch with your feet in different positions (stride, straddle, together)?
2. catch while standing straight?
3. catch from a crouched position?
4. catch from a squatting position?
5. catch from a kneeling position?
6. catch while sitting?
7. find different body positions in which to catch the ball?
8. catch while looking forward?
9. catch while looking at the ball?
10. catch with your eyes closed?
11. catch a slow-moving ball?

12. catch a fast-moving ball?
13. catch a high, arching ball?
14. catch a high ball?
15. catch a knee high ball?
16. catch an ankle high ball?
17. catch a ball tossed to your right side? Left side?
18. turn and catch a ball?
19. catch a bounced ball?
20. catch a ball coming straight down?
21. catch with other body parts?
22. catch with your hands and arms?
23. catch with your hands only?
24. catch with your palms facing each other?
25. catch progressively smaller balls?

Challenge Activities with Small Balls

Many of the activities with the large ball may be repeated with a small ball, which may be made out of newspaper, sponge, or rubber.

Can you . . .

1. catch with both hands at the ankles, knees, hips, chest, shoulders, or head?
2. catch with both hands and emphasize the arm action by catching with your arms straight? With your arms bent? With your arms straight, then bringing the object close to your body?
3. catch an object that is thrown to the left or right side of your body at various heights?
4. attempt to catch with one hand a ball that is rolled, bounced, or thrown at various heights?
5. toss the ball upward and catch it?
6. find different ways to toss the ball to yourself and catch it?
7. play toss and catch with a partner?
8. catch a ball thrown at different heights?
9. catch a ball thrown at different speeds?
10. catch a ball thrown from different directions?
11. catch a ball thrown in different arcs?
12. catch with one hand?
13. catch with the other hand?
14. run and catch?
15. jump in the air and catch?

KICKING

In kicking, the foot imparts force to objects. A movement pattern often poorly developed in American youth, it is described in detail in Chapter 4.

The following developmental and remedial activities are designed to improve both kicking and trapping (stopping).

Challenge Activities to Develop Kicking Abilities

Can you . . .

1. kick with your toe?
2. kick with your instep?
3. kick with the inside of your foot?
4. kick with the outside of your foot?
5. kick with your heel?
6. kick as hard as you can?
7. kick as easily as you can?
8. kick as far as you can?
9. kick at a target?
10. kick to a partner?
11. kick between objects?
12. kick in a straight line?
13. drop the ball and kick it before it hits the ground?
14. kick a rolling ball?
15. kick a ball rolling to you?
16. kick a ball rolling away from you?
17. kick a bouncing ball?
18. kick a football (soccer ball, Wiffle ball, tennis ball, and so on)?
19. kick and keep the ball on the ground?
20. kick the ball into the air?

Challenge Activities to Develop Trapping Abilities

Can you . . .

1. trap the ball with the sole of your foot?
2. trap the ball with your shins?
3. trap the ball with one knee?
4. trap the ball with your stomach?
5. trap the ball with your bottom?
6. trap the ball with your arms?
7. trap the ball on your knees?
8. trap the ball from a crab position?
9. trap different-sized balls?
10. trap the ball while seated?
11. trap balls traveling at different speeds?
12. trap a bouncing ball?
13. trap a ball coming from different directions?

REMEDIAL MOVEMENT EXPERIENCES

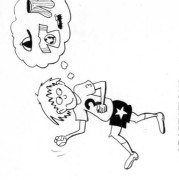

Throwing

The following remedial movement experiences are designed to improve specific body actions of the throwing pattern. Children should be given the opportunity to develop mature arm, trunk, and leg-foot actions.

POINTS TO EMPHASIZE	MOVEMENT EXPERIENCES	ADAPTATIONS
	Distance Throw	
Step, shift in weight; correct arm action; complete follow-through.	Have each child throw a small ball as far as possible. Mark each child's farthest throw and have him or her break his or her own record. Stress the form of the throw as well as the power.	1. Have the children throw the ball while keeping their feet stationary. 2. Tell the children to toss the ball with the non-throwing hand. 3. Have the children run and throw the ball.
	Step and Throw	
Step, shift in weight; trunk action.	Have the children practice stepping out and throwing a ball against a wall. Throwers should stand behind a line, step forward while throwing, and complete the throwing action in front of the line.	1. Instruct the children to vary the throwing pattern: overhand, underhand, sidearm, or two-handed throw from chest level. 2. Mark a target on the wall and have the children attempt to hit it. Keep score. 3. Increase the distance from the wall.

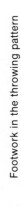

Footwork in the throwing pattern

187

POINTS TO EMPHASIZE

Arm action centered at elbow, accurate release of object, complete follow-through.

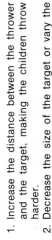

Correct action of nondominant foot, trunk rotation, overhand throwing pattern.

MOVEMENT EXPERIENCES

Target Throw

Construct targets of various sizes and shapes. Have the children stand behind a line and attempt to throw balls and beanbags of various sizes and shapes at the target.

From the Stretch

Have the children stand with their nonthrowing side toward the target or wall. The ball should be held in front of the body with the arms relaxed. When ready, the child should step toward the target with the nondominant foot as the throwing arm prepares for the throw. The elbow should lead the throwing action, and there should be a complete follow-through. It may be helpful to lay out the following foot pattern to aid children who are experiencing difficulty.

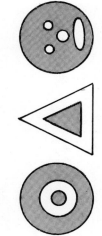

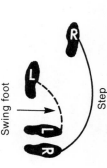

Swing foot

Step

ADAPTATIONS

1. Instruct the children to move further from the target, to move at an angle, or to decrease the size of the target.
2. Suspend a target and have the children attempt to toss the ball through a swinging target.

1. Increase the distance between the thrower and the target, making the children throw harder.
2. Decrease the size of the target or vary the size of the ball or both.
3. Have the children throw without benefit of the foot pattern.
4. Tell the children to make believe they are pitching to a batter; can they throw three strikes before they walk the imaginary batter?

POINTS TO EMPHASIZE	MOVEMENT EXPERIENCES	ADAPTATIONS

Rapid Fire

Use of the correct pattern when rapidly performing movement, shift in weight on opposite foot.

The children stand on a line and take turns tossing the ball to the instructor, who is standing directly in front of them. Once the children catch the ball, they should throw the ball back without delay, using a mature throwing pattern.

1. Increase the distance between the instructor and the children.
2. Utilize balls, beanbags, and other objects of various shapes and sizes.
3. Have the children vary the type of throw used to return the ball: underhand, overhand, bounce, chest, and so on.
4. Vary the throwing pattern used.

Pitcher

Complete pattern: step, shift in weight, hip snap, elbow lead, complete follow-through.

On a wall mark a square box approximately the size of a strike zone. Cut a batting plate out of poster board and place it on the floor. The children should pitch from a line that has been marked on the floor. Instruct the children to strike out the batter instead of walking him. Keep score of how many runs are walked before three outs are made.

1. Increase the distance from the plate to the pitcher's mound.
2. Have a catcher call balls and strikes.
3. Using a plastic ball and bat, play a modified game of baseball.

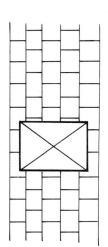

189

Catching

The following remedial activities should enhance the ability to catch a thrown object. Children should especially work on visual perception and arm and hand position.

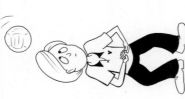

POINTS TO EMPHASIZE

Keep eyes on balloon, fingers control balloon.

Finger control, correct hand position (little fingers in opposition).

MOVEMENT EXPERIENCES

Balloon Catch

Give each child a previously inflated balloon. Explore with the children the various ways in which the balloon can be tossed into the air and caught.

Ground Ball

Have the children pick partners and stand approximately 10 feet apart facing each other. Give one child of each pair a large playground ball and tell him or her to roll it to the partner. The "fielder" should be positioned in front of the ball and should pick it up with the fingers. Initially have the children stand and roll the ball. Then instruct them to catch the ball; with success they should move forward and attempt to control the ball.

ADAPTATIONS

1. Instruct the children to pair off and play catch with the balloon.
2. Have the children use balloons of various shapes and sizes.

1. Vary the size of the ball from a large playground ball to a small tennis ball.
2. Roll the ball to the left and right of the fielder.
3. Roll the ball with a slight bounce to the fielder.

POINTS TO EMPHASIZE	MOVEMENT EXPERIENCES	ADAPTATIONS
	Bounce and Catch	
Good absorption of momentum of bounced ball, use of fingers, eyes on ball.	Partners should face each other with a hoop placed on the floor between them. With a large playground ball, one child should attempt a chest pass (stepping off the nondominant foot) into the hoop and thereby bounce it to the catcher. Repeat.	1. Vary the size of the ball from a large playground ball to a small tennis ball. 2. Place the hoop in various positions. How does that affect the bounce?
	Beanbag Catch	
Keep eyes on beanbag; catch it with the fingers.	Make beanbags of various shapes such as geometric forms, letters, or numbers. Have children select partners and stand a few feet apart. Give one child of each pair a sack filled with several beanbags of different shapes. The thrower should select a beanbag without letting the catcher see it and then should toss it high into the air. The other child should attempt to identify the shape before he or she catches it.	1. Decrease the height that the beanbag is tossed into the air. 2. Add more difficult shapes to each sack of beanbags. 3. Have the children toss beanbags using various movement patterns.

POINTS TO EMPHASIZE	MOVEMENT EXPERIENCES	ADAPTATIONS

Control the ball; adjust to the flight of the ball.

Individual Ball Activities

Instruct the children to find a space on the floor and give each a hoop and a large playground ball. Have students place the hoop on the floor and while standing outside the hoop:

A. Bounce the ball in the hoop and catch it with both hands, one hand, and then no hands.

B. Toss the ball various heights into the air, let it bounce in the hoop, and then catch it with one or both hands.

C. Toss the ball high into the air. Clap hands as often as possible before catching the ball after it bounces.

D. Do the same as in "C", but attempt to make complete turns before having to catch the ball.

E. Toss the ball various heights and catch it before it bounces; don't leave the hoop.

F. Toss the ball into the air; turn and catch it before it bounces.

G. Toss the ball into the air; clap hands and attempt to catch it before it bounces.

1. Vary the size of the ball, progressing from large to small.

2. Instead of a hoop, use boxes of various sizes or ropes.

Correct arm position, eyes on ball; finger control.

Circle Catch

Have the children form a circle, facing a catcher who has been selected to stand in the center. Using proper form, the children on the circumference of the circle should toss a ball to the catcher. The child in the center should catch the ball with the fingers, turn to the next child, throw, and then receive a returned toss. After the child has made a complete circle, another child should be selected as catcher.

1. Vary the direction in which the catcher turns around the circle.

2. Vary the size and shape of the ball or beanbag.

3. Vary the type of throw utilized: underhand, overhand, bounce, chest, and so on.

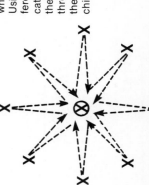

Kicking

The following remedial activities are designed to improve children's ability to perform a mature kicking pattern.

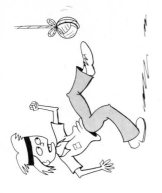

POINTS TO EMPHASIZE	MOVEMENT EXPERIENCES	ADAPTATIONS
Balance maintained, leg swings from hip, complete follow-through.	*Stationary Kick* Have the children place a large playground ball approximately one step from them. They should then attempt to kick the ball as hard as possible, utilizing a mature kicking form. If the children have difficulty maintaining balance, have them hold onto a stationary object, such as a chair or a partner, while kicking. A diagrammed foot pattern may prove helpful.	1. Vary the size of the ball, progressing from large to small. 2. Have the children utilize various parts of the foot, such as the instep or the toe, while attempting to kick. 3. Tell the children to stand farther from the ball and take several steps before kicking it.
Arms in position.	*Arm Swing* As the children perform a kicking pattern, have them hold a small weighted object in each hand. First, have the children practice swinging their kicking leg and working their arms in opposition. After some practice, instruct the children to hold the weights while kicking the ball.	1. Vary the weights of the objects held by the children. 2. Have the children hold the weighted object in their nondominant hand and be sure that this hand is forward at contact. 3. Have the children hold weighted objects and then stand and kick a stationary and a rolled ball; they should then run and kick a stationary and rolled ball.

POINTS TO EMPHASIZE

Eyes on ball.

MOVEMENT EXPERIENCES

Kick and Look

Cut out of poster board a series of small circles. On each, draw a number or letter large enough to be seen easily from a distance of approximately 5 feet. Fold a piece of masking tape on the back of each cut-out so that it will stick to the floor. Before each kick, a cut-out should be placed under the ball without the kicker seeing the letter or number that has been drawn on it. The ball should be slightly deflated so that it will completely cover the cut-out. As the kicker kicks the ball as hard as possible, he or she should call out the number or letter drawn on the cut-out.

ADAPTATIONS

1. Have the children try to kick the ball with their eyes closed.
2. Use various numbers, letters, colors, and shapes for the child to identify.
3. Have the children attempt to run, kick the ball, and identify the cut-out.

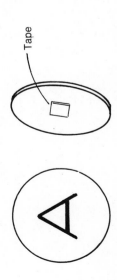

Tape

POINTS TO EMPHASIZE	MOVEMENT EXPERIENCES	ADAPTATIONS
	Kicking a Rolled Ball	
Arms in opposition, leg swings from hip, correct foot position.	Have the children kick a ball that is rolled to them. Children should initially kick une ball from a stationary position and then attempt to kick it while running.	1. Vary the size of the kicked ball. 2. Vary the speed of the rolled ball. 3. Have the children try to kick a ball that is rolled first to their left and then to their right. 4. Have the children attempt to kick a ball that is rolled with a slight bounce.
	Punting	
Leg swings from hip, complete follow-through.	Have the children stand with weight evenly distributed and hold a ball with both hands in front of the body. Children should simultaneously drop the ball and swing the kicking leg to make contact. The follow-through of the kicking leg should be high while maintaining balance.	1. Use balls of various sizes and shapes; balloons are particularly helpful for children having difficulty coordinating the kicking action. 2. Have children attempt to punt a ball to a partner or target.
	High Rise	
Complete, high follow-through.	Suspend a large ball on a rope at approximately waist height. Instruct the children to take one step and simulate kicking the suspended ball and following through.	1. Raise the height of the suspended ball. 2. Have the children actually attempt to kick the ball and complete the follow-through.

MOVEMENT EXPERIENCES DESIGNED TO ENHANCE SUPPLEMENTAL MANIPULATIVE PATTERNS

STRIKING

The development of the striking pattern has not been extensively researched and thus is a fertile area for serious study. Samples of striking activities appropriate for preschool and primary grade children follow.

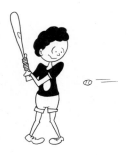

See if you can . . .

1. strike an object with one hand or an implement held by one hand while standing with the feet in a stride or straddle position and either close together or far apart.
2. repeat the action in number 1, using two hands or an implement held with two hands.
3. use the underhand, sidearm, or overhand pattern with one or both hands to strike an object.
4. use the underhand, sidearm, or overhand striking pattern while standing, kneeling, sitting, or lying.
5. lean the trunk forward, backward, and sideward when using the different striking patterns.
6. strike a stationary, resting, rolling, or airborne object lightly, firmly, slowly, or quickly.
7. strike an object and emphasize the follow-through beyond the point of contact.
8. strike an object so that the point of contact and the transfer of weight are timed to a verbal cue or drum beat.
9. strike an object rolling on the floor or airborne at different heights with one or both hands or with an implement.
10. strike a stationary or resting object with short jabs or large sweeping movements.
11. strike an object from above or below, from the right or left, and from other angles.

12. strike a rolling object with the hand as you walk or run alongside it.
13. strike an airborne object and skip to retrieve it.
14. strike a stationary object on a tee with an implement while balancing on one foot.
15. use a short striking action and roll or slide an object along a bench or balance beam.
16. use an implement to strike a vertical or horizontal pole with colored targets.
17. strike an object, such as a balloon or feather, into the air and catch it.

BOUNCING

Bouncing a ball requires considerable eye-hand coordination and may incorporate dribbling. The following list is a sampling of bouncing activities suitable for young children.

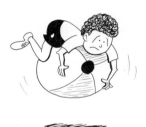

Can you . . .

1. bounce and catch the ball while standing?
2. bounce and catch the ball while sitting?
3. bounce and catch the ball while kneeling?
4. bounce and catch the ball while squatting?
5. bounce and catch the ball while bent forward?
6. bounce and catch the ball while on your toes?
7. bounce and catch the ball in different positions?
8. bounce the ball at different heights (high, low, or medium)?
9. bounce and clap?
10. bounce and turn?
11. bounce and make a funny face?
12. bounce and catch with one hand?
13. bounce and catch with other body parts?
14. bounce and catch to music?
15. bounce and catch with a partner?

16. bounce and catch against a wall?
17. bounce and catch while walking in different directions (forward, backward, and so on)?
18. bounce and catch with your eyes closed?
19. bounce and catch while walking, running, jumping, or galloping?
20. dribble the ball?
21. dribble in a limited area?
22. dribble in place?
23. dribble with each hand?
24. change hands while dribbling?
25. look up while dribbling?
26. dribble while walking forward, backward, or sideward?
27. dribble among other children?
28. dribble between objects?
29. dribble, circling your body?
30. dribble as long as you can?
31. dribble as fast or slowly as you can?
32. dribble as high or low as you can?
33. dribble while running?

ROLLING

Rolling, one of the first propulsive movements learned by the infant, involves imparting force to an object along a flat surface. A list of some rolling activities appropriate for young children follows.

Can you . . .

1. roll the ball from a seated straddle position?
2. roll the ball from a crosslegged position?
3. roll the ball from a position on your knees?
4. roll the ball from a squat position?
5. roll the ball from a standing straddle position?
6. roll the ball from a standing stride position?
7. roll the ball around your body while lying on the floor?
8. roll at a target while sitting, kneeling, standing, or in a seated straddle position?
9. roll softly, smoothly, quickly, slowly, forcefully, or at an angle?
10. initiate rolling movements at the sound of a hand clap, drum beat, or records?
11. roll against a wall, between two boxes, toward an Indian club, over an incline board, or under a wicket?
12. roll on the floor, on a bench, on a beam, and down a slide?
13. toss the ball in the air, let it bounce, catch it, and roll it into a box?
14. pretend the object you are rolling is very heavy or very light?
15. roll a cageball, basketball, playground ball, soccer ball, softball, Wiffle ball, tennis ball, baseball, ping pong ball, or marble?

16. roll an object on a hard floor, on a mat, up or down an incline board, over a maze of ropes, or on grass or dirt surfaces outside?

SUMMARY

This chapter has presented a wide variety of sample developmental and remedial movement activities for refining fundamental manipulative abilities. The experiences are designed to stimulate interest and encourage practice in various manipulative movements. Since *fun* is the key to effective learning by children, movement activities have to be both fun and challenging to be of any real merit. The teacher is encouraged to go beyond the ideas presented here and to structure movement experiences geared specifically to the needs, interests, and ability level of the particular children involved.

BIBLIOGRAPHY

1. Anderson, Marion, Elliot, Margaret E., and LaBerge, Jeanne: *Play with a Purpose.* New York: Harper and Row, 1972.
2. Brown, Margaret G., and Sommer, Betty: *Movement Education: Its Evolution and a Modern Approach.* Reading, Mass.: Addison-Wesley, 1969.
3. Dauer, Victor P.: *Essential Movement Experiences for Pre school and Primary Grade Children.* Minneapolis: Burgess, 1971.
4. Frostig, Marianne, and Maslow, Phyliss: *Movement Education: Theory and Practice.* Chicago: Follett, 1970.
5. Gallahue, David: *Motor Development and Movement Experiences for Young Children (3–7).* New York: John Wiley, 1976.
6. Gilliom, Bonnie: *Basic Movement Education for Children.* Reading, Mass.: Addison-Wesley, 1970.
7. Hackett, Layne C., and Jenson, Robert G.: *A Guide to Movement Exploration.* Palo Alto, Calif.: Peek Publications, 1967.
8. Logsdon, Bette J., and Barrett, Kate R.: *Ready? Set . . . Go!* Bloomington, Ind.: National Instructional Television, 1970.
9. Schurr, Evelyn: *Movement Experiences for Children.* Englewood Cliffs, N.J.: Prentice-Hall, 1975.

APPENDIX A
Supplemental Reading List

Section 1: Fundamental Movement

Arnheim, Daniel D., and Sinclair, William A.: *The Clumsy Child: A Program of Motor Therapy.* St. Louis: C. V. Mosby Co., 1975.

Beter, Thais R., and Cragin, Wesley: *The Mentally Retarded Child and His Motor Behavior.* Springfield, Ill.: Charles C Thomas, 1972.

Connolly, K. J.: *Mechanisms of Motor Skill Development.* New York: Academic Press.

Corbin, Charles: *A Textbook of Motor Development.* Dubuque, Iowa: William C. Brown, 1973.

Cratty, Bryant J.: *Perceptual and Motor Development of Infants and Children.* New York: Macmillan, 1972.

Cratty, Bryant J.: *Remedial Motor Activity for Children.* Philadelphia: Lea and Febiger, 1975.

Espenschade, Anna S., and Eckert, Helen M.: *Motor Development.* Columbus, Ohio: Charles E. Merrill, 1967.

Flinchmin, Betty: *Motor Development in Early Childhood.* St. Louis: C. V. Mosby Co., 1975.

Gallahue, David L.: *Motor Development and Movement Experiences for Young Children.* New York: John Wiley, 1976.

Gallahue, David L., Werner, Peter H., and Luedke, George C.: *A Conceptual Approach to Moving and Learning.* New York: John Wiley, 1975.

Halverson, Lolas: The young child . . . the significance of motor development. *The Significance of the Child's Motor Development.* Washington, D.C.: National Association of Young Children, 1971.

Rarick, G. Lawrence (ed.): *Physical Activity: Human Growth and Development.* New York: Academic Press, 1973.

Stelmalh, George E. (ed.): *Motor Control: Issues and Trends.* New York: Academic Press, 1976.

Whitenhurst, Keturah: The young child . . . what movement means to him. *The Significance of the Young Child's Motor Development.* Washington, D.C.: National Association for the Education of Young Children, 1971.

Wickstrom, Ralph: *Fundamental Motor Patterns.* Philadelphia: Lea and Febiger, 1977.

Section 2: Program Design

Corbin, Charles B.: *Becoming Physically Educated in the Elementary School.* Philadelphia: Lea and Febiger, 1976.

Halverson, Lolas: Development of motor patterns in young children. *Quest. VI, A Symposium on Motor Learning,* 6:44–53, 1966.

Kraus, Richard: *Therapeutic Recreation Services.* Philadelphia: W. B. Saunders Co., 1972.

Kruger, Hayes, and Kruger, Jane M.: *Movement Education in Physical Education: A Guide to Teaching and Planning.* Dubuque, Iowa: William C. Brown, 1977.

Logsdon, Bette J., et al.: *Physical Education for Children: A Focus on the Teaching Process.* Philadelphia: Lea and Febiger, 1977.

Mager, Robert: *Preparing Instructional Objectives.* Belmont, Calif.: Fearon Publishers, 1975.

Popham, James W., and Baker, Eva I.: *Systematic Instruction.* Englewood Cliffs, N.J.: Prentice-Hall, 1971.

Tyler, Ralph: *Basic Principles of Curriculum and Instruction.* Chicago: University of Chicago Press, 1971.

Section 3: Movement Experiences

Arnheim, Daniel D., and Sinclair, William A.: *The Clumsy Child: A Program of Motor Therapy.* St. Louis: C. V. Mosby Co., 1975.

Block, Susan: *Me—I Am Great: Physical Education for Children Three Through Eight.* Minneapolis: Burgess, 1977.

Cratty, Bryant J.: *Remedial Motor Activity for Children.* Philadelphia: Lea and Febiger, 1975.

Dauer, Victor P., and Pangrazi, Robert P.: *Dynamic Physical Education for Elementary School Children.* Minneapolis: Burgess, 1975.

Gallahue, David L.: *Motor Development and Movement Experiences for Young Children.* New York: John Wiley, 1976.

Gallahue, David L., Werner, Peter H., and Luedke, George C.: *A Conceptual Approach to Moving and Learning.* New York: John Wiley, 1975.

Hall, Tillman, et al.: *Until the Whistle Blows.* Santa Monica, Calif.: Goodyear Publishing, 1976.

Kirchner, Glen: *Physical Education for Elementary School Children.* Dubuque, Iowa: William C. Brown, 1970.

Moran, Joan M., and Kalakian, Leonard H.: *Movement Experiences for Mentally Retarded and Emotionally Disturbed Children.* Minneapolis: Burgess, 1977.

Morris, Don: *How to Change the Games Children Play.* Minneapolis: Burgess, 1976.

Schurr, Evelyn: *Movement Experiences for Children.* Englewood Cliffs, N.J.: Prentice-Hall, 1975.

Vannier, MaryHelen, and Gallahue, David L.: *Teaching Physical Education in Elementary Schools.* Philadelphia: W. B. Saunders Co., 1978.

APPENDIX B

Examples of Inexpensive Equipment for Enhancing Fundamental Movement

Equipment	Materials	Approximate Cost
1. Ropes of various lengths	200 feet of rope, tape for both ends	$14.00
2. Hoops of various sizes	$\frac{1}{2}$- to $\frac{3}{4}$-inch plastic pipe, wooden dowels, tape	.65 per hoop
3. Carpet squares	Extra carpet or samples	Free
4. Beanbags of various sizes and shapes	Cloth, thread, popcorn, or filler	$.15 per bag
5. Yarn balls	Skein of yarn	$.85 per skein
6. Bamboo poles	Centers of carpet rolls	Free
7. Bouncing tubes	Auto inner tubes	Free
8. Stretch tubes	Bicycle inner tubes or cut auto tubes	Free
9. Wands (Lumi sticks)	Wooden dowels or cut broom handles	$.75 per 3-foot dowel
10. Can stilts	Tin cans, rope, tape, or plastic lid	Free
11. Balance boards	$\frac{3}{4}$- inch plywood, 2-foot × 4-foot blocks	$10.00

12. Balance beam	4-foot × 4-foot board, two 2-foot × 4-foot boards for legs	$15.00 each
13. Barrels	Old barrels, cleaned	$5.00 each
14. Bowling pins	Small plastic bottles	Free
15. Catching scoops	Large plastic bottles, tape	Free
16. Hockey set	Old brooms, paper ball	Free

The reader interested in inexpensive equipment may find the following texts helpful:

Christian, Quentin A.: *The Bean Bag Curriculum: A Homemade Approach to Physical Activity for Children.* Wolfe City, Texas: The University Press, 1973.

Corbin, Charles B.: *Inexpensive Equipment for Games, Play and Physical Activity.* Dubuque, Iowa: William C. Brown, 1972.

Gallahue, David L.: *Developmental Play Equipment for Home and School.* New York: John Wiley, 1975.

Werner, Peter, and Rini, Lisa: *Perceptual Motor Development Equipment.* New York: John Wiley, 1976.

Werner, Peter, and Simmons, Richard: *Inexpensive Physical Education Equipment for Children.* Minneapolis: Burgess, 1976.

The following is a list of commercial suppliers of equipment for motor development programs.

Cosom Corporation
6030 Wayzata Boulevard
Minneapolis, Minnesota 55416

Creative Playthings
A Division of Columbia Broadcasting System, Inc.
Princeton, New Jersey 08540

Developmental Learning Materials
7440 Natchez Avenue
Niles, Illinois 60648

Ed-Nu, Inc.
5115 Route 38
Pennsauken, New Jersey 08109

Educational Activities, Inc.
P.O. Box 392
Freeport, New York 11520

Flaghouse, Inc.
18 West 18th Street
New York, New York 10011

Gym-thing
19 West Pennsylvania Avenue
Towson, Maryland 21204

J. L. Hammett Co.
2393 Vaux Hall Road
Union, New Jersey 07083

The Delmer F. Harris Co.
Concordia, Kansas 66901

Ideal School Supply Co.
11000 S. Lavergne Avenue
Oak Lawn, Illinois 60453

Jayfro Corporation
P.O. Box 400
Waterford, Connecticut 06385

Hoctor Dance Records, Inc.
Waldwick, New Jersey 07463

Milton Bradley Co.
Springfield, Massachusetts 01101

Passon's, Inc.
824 Arch Street
Philadelphia, Pennsylvania 19107

J. A. Preston Corporation
71 Fifth Avenue
New York, New York 10003

Skill Development Equipment Co.
1340 North Jefferson
Anaheim, California 92806

Snitz Sports Supply Co.
104 South Church Street
East Troy, Wisconsin 53120

Teaching Resources Corporation
100 Boylston Street
Boston, Massachusetts 02116

Things From Bell, Inc.
P.O. Box 26
90 Clinton Street
Homer, New York 13077

Vantel Corporation
P.O. Box 6590
Orange, California 92667

W. J. Voit Rubber Corporation
29 Essex Street
Maywood, New Jersey 07607

Wolverine Sports
745 State Circle
Ann Arbor, Michigan 48104

Wilson Sporting Goods Co.
2233 West Street
River Grove, Illinois 60171

World Publications
P.O. Box 366
Mountain View, California 94040

APPENDIX C
Developmental Playgrounds

The reader may have the opportunity to plan a developmental playground that is designed to improve children's physical abilities and fundamental movement abilities. The following is a list of companies that manufacture playground equipment.

Big Toys and Growing Big Toys
Northwest Design Products, Inc.
Tacoma, Washington 98409

Childscapes, Inc.
6487 Peachtree Industrial Blvd.
Atlanta, Georgia 30360

Creative Playgrounds Corporation
R.R. 23-1234 East 99 Drive
Terre Haute, Indiana 47802

Game Time, Inc.
900 Anderson Road
Litchfield, Michigan 49252

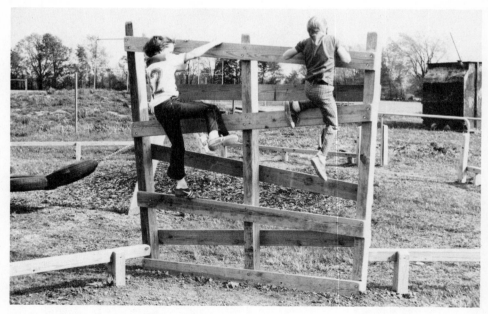

Children on a developmental playground. (Courtesy of Creative Playgrounds Corp., Terre Haute, Ind. Used with permission.)

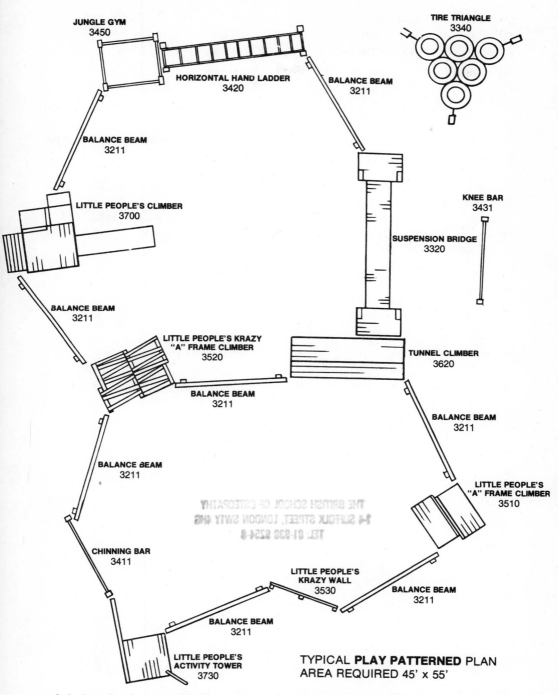

TYPICAL **PLAY PATTERNED** PLAN
AREA REQUIRED 45' x 55'

A design of a playground that is constructed from treated lumber. Children can move from one piece of equipment to the next without touching the ground. Individuals can contact commercial companies that offer numerous designs to meet particular needs. (Courtesy of Creative Playgrounds Corp., Terre Haute, Ind. Used with permission.)

Landscape Structures, Inc.
300 Dawn Heather Drive
Delanco, Minnesota 55328

Northwest Design Products, Inc.
1235 South Tacoma Way
Tacoma, Washington 98409

Mexico Forge
P.O. Box 565
Reedsville, Pennsylvania 17084

Timberform
1975 S.W. Fifth Avenue
Portland, Oregon 97201

The following texts may provide the reader with additional information on constructing playgrounds.

Friedberg, M. Paul: *Handcrafted Playgrounds: Designs You Can Build Yourself.* New York: Random House, 1975.
Hogan, Paul: *Playgrounds For Free.* Cambridge, Mass.: MIT Press, 1974.
Miller, Peggy L.: *Creative Outdoor Play Areas.* Englewood Cliffs, N.J.: Prentice-Hall, 1972.

INDEX